Origins of the Human Mind
Part II

Professor Stephen P. Hinshaw

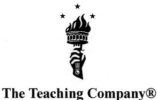

The Teaching Company®

PUBLISHED BY:

THE TEACHING COMPANY
4840 Westfields Boulevard, Suite 500
Chantilly, Virginia 20151-2299
1-800-TEACH-12
Fax—703-378-3819
www.teach12.com

ISBN 1-59803-638-6

Stephen P. Hinshaw, Ph.D.

Professor of Psychology
and Chair of the Department of Psychology
University of California, Berkeley

Professor Stephen P. Hinshaw is Professor and Chair of the Department of Psychology at the University of California, Berkeley. After receiving his A.B. summa cum laude from Harvard University in 1974, he directed day school and residential programs for children with developmental disabilities for 3 years. In 1983, he received his Ph.D. in Clinical Psychology from the University of California, Los Angeles; in 1980, he received the UCLA alumni association's Distinguished Scholar Award, which honors the university's outstanding graduate student.

Professor Hinshaw was a clinical psychology intern at UCLA's Neuropsychiatric Institute from 1981 to 1982. He then was a postdoctoral fellow at the Langley Porter Psychiatric Institute of the University of California, San Francisco, from 1983 to 1985, where he received the Robert E. Harris Award. He taught in the Psychology Department at UCLA from 1986 to 1990 and joined the UC Berkeley faculty in 1990. He received the Distinguished Teaching Award from UC Berkeley's Division of Social Sciences, College of Letters and Science, in 2001.

Professor Hinshaw's work focuses on developmental psychopathology, with particular emphases on peer and family relationships in children with externalizing disorders, neuropsychological risk factors for and correlates of psychopathology, comparisons and combinations of pharmacological and psychological interventions for children with attention deficit/hyperactivity disorder (ADHD), assessment and evaluation, conceptual and definitional issues in the field, and the stigmatization of mental illness. For more than 25 years, he has directed summer research camps for, and conducted longitudinal studies of, boys (and more recently, girls) with ADHD and associated disorders.

Professor Hinshaw is the editor of *Psychological Bulletin*, the most cited journal in the entire field of psychology. He is also an associate editor of the journal *Development and Psychopathology* and has authored more than 200 articles, chapters, and reviews on child psychopathology. His first book was *Attention Deficits and Hyperactivity in Children* (Sage, 1994). His other books include *The Years of Silence Are Past: My Father's Life with Bipolar Disorder* (Cambridge University Press, 2002) and *The Mark of Shame: Stigma of Mental Illness and an Agenda for Change* (Oxford University Press, 2007). Professor Hinshaw's edited books include *Breaking the Silence: Mental Health Professionals Disclose Their Personal and Family Experiences of Mental Illness* (Oxford University Press, 2008) and *Child and Adolescent Psychopathology* (Wiley, 2008), coedited with Theodore P. Beauchaine. His newest book is *The Triple Bind: Saving Our Teenage Girls from Today's Pressures* (Random House/ Ballantine, 2009), coauthored with Rachel Kranz.

In support of his research efforts, Professor Hinshaw has received more than $13 million in grants from the National Institute of Mental Health and other federal agencies. He is past president of the International Society for Research in Child and Adolescent Psychopathology and Division 53 of the American Psychological Association (Society for Clinical Child and Adolescent Psychology). He is also a Fellow of the Association For Psychological Science, the American Psychological Association, and the American Association for the Advancement of Science.

Professor Hinshaw lives in Berkeley, California, with his wife, Kelly Campbell Hinshaw, an art educator and children's book author. They have 3 sons.

Table of Contents
Origins of the Human Mind
Part II

Origins of the Human Mind

Scope:

Among the animal kingdom, the human mind is the only one to reflect on its own nature and development. Our minds are unsurpassed in flexibility, imagination, creativity, and narrative ability, but they are also subject to distortions and biases as well as the potential for highly impairing mental disturbances. Modern neuroscience has shifted the view of our minds—as inextricably linked to complex brain chemistry rather than the products of spirits or supernatural forces—with major implications for how we perceive ourselves as a species. The emergence of our minds from non-human minds, their development across each human lifespan and their linkages with brain functions, whether they are modular or general purpose in nature, how they are shaped by contextual factors, and how they can both flourish and "go wrong": These are the core issues addressed in this course.

A number of perplexing questions continue to be addressed by philosophers, biologists, psychologists, and neuroscientists: How have the unique aspects of the human brain and human mind evolved from those of mammals and primates? Have they continued to develop across our species' time on Earth? What are the implications of natural selection and modern brain science for understanding our minds and ourselves? How have humans viewed their own minds throughout history? What roles do temperament, attachments with caregivers, family childrearing styles, neighborhoods, and culture play in forming each of our behavioral and emotional styles? In what ways can the mind go awry as we experience trauma or suffer from mental disturbance? Are we fundamentally prosocial or aggressive as a species? Can we create a more humane view of all individuals by acknowledging our diversity and using our narrative abilities to humanize our peers? These questions and more are addressed.

Modern neuroscience informs us that we are born with over 100 billion neurons, meaning that several thousand new neurons are created during each and every second of our 40 weeks in the womb. Across the first years of life, these neurons develop elaborate networks of interconnection with one another, linking at synapses. Through processes of pruning, neurons that do not form such connections are lost, creating a more efficient mind. Genes are clearly involved in shaping neural connections and in pruning, but life experiences activate genes and forge how and where neurons interconnect. In short, brain development is marked by plasticity—and evolution clearly favored human minds with the ability to be molded by experience. Because our brains and minds are involved in an elaborate interplay of biology and contextual forces, we must traverse multiple levels of analysis, from genes to families and cultures, to gain deep understanding.

An introductory lecture provides the course framework, emphasizing spirit-based, naturalistic, and humanistic models for understanding the mind. Next, we cover the structure and function of the brain, with much attention given to principles of brain development. Evolution is the next focus, followed by core psychological views of the mind: psychodynamic theory, from Freud to modern psychoanalytic concepts, and social learning theory from Pavlov, Skinner, and Watson to the modern cognitive behaviorists. The progression across evolutionary development from instinct to learning is featured, along with the modularity of the mind's functioning and information about the cognitive revolution and emotion revolution of the last century. We next consider recent microevolutionary investigations, which emphasize that the core difference between human brains and those of primates is not sheer size but the number of neurons in the cortex and the massive, high-speed interconnections across brain regions. Human evolution favored brains with great responsiveness to our complex social environments.

Individual development is covered in the next set of lectures, from the earliest years of childhood through adolescence, adulthood, and aging. Key topics include temperament, attachment, and the contextual factors of families, neighborhoods, and culture. Important questions include whether adolescent minds are inevitably rebellious and whether the advancing years signal inevitable decline versus the development of wisdom. Subsequent lectures deal with gender and the mind, risk and protective factors, and interactions between biology and experience.

We then address the building blocks of life—genes and DNA—and the concepts of heritability and gene-environment interplay to explain individual differences in human minds. Because recent science emphasizes that genes and environments work in concert in incredible ways, the dichotomy of nature versus nurture is sorely out of date. We then discuss how minds are altered by trauma and mental illness.

Indeed, when positive features of the mind are thwarted, mental disorders—such as post-traumatic reactions, schizophrenia, mood disorders, disruptions of attention and regulation, and autism—may result. Such conditions inform us about the mind's ultimate potential. From an evolutionary perspective it is not deviant genes but rather mismatches between our genetic heritage and the nature of our current human environments that underlie disordered functioning.

Considered next is how evolution has shaped our human tendencies to be religious, to show aggression versus prosocial behavior, and to stigmatize fellow humans who are not members of our primary ingroups. Personal and family narratives, which exemplify the mythic skills of all humans, offer a key means of humanizing one another. The final lecture includes advances in the study of the human brain and mind, with implications for renewed self-understanding.

Spanning historical models, evolutionary and microevolutionary forces, links between biology and experience, the role of development, the arena of mental disturbance, and the potential for emergence of a more humane view of the varieties of human behavior, this course provides a tour of fundamental questions in psychology, psychiatry, evolution, neuroscience, narrative, and ethics.

Lecture Thirteen
Parallels between Development and Evolution

Scope:

A major question regarding both individual development and evolutionary development is whether they operate continuously and smoothly versus discontinuously, or in stages. Although the answer depends largely on the scale of measurement, discontinuous shifts in both individual development and the development of species are quite apparent. Regarding the development of humans, risk factors are variables within the person or environment that precede and predict negative outcomes. Some are fixed and some are malleable; the premium is on finding truly causal risk factors that can be altered. We therefore explore protective factors, which promote healthy outcome and resilient functioning despite high probabilities of maladaptation.

Outline

I. Environmental and biological factors operate reciprocally and transactionally in both individual development and evolution by natural selection.

   A. It is not just that influences work together; they do so by repeated patterns of reciprocal influence. When such reciprocal influences repeat themselves over time, we say that the process is transactional.

   B. Transactional processes also characterize evolution. A mutation may induce a behavior change that is adaptive in a certain environment; the environment then produces selection pressure favoring reproduction for those individuals with the mutation and its new behavior patterns.

   C. Co-evolution occurs when changes in one species influence changes in another.

II. Does development occur smoothly and continuously, or discontinuously and in stages? In some ways, this is a trick question: whether a graph of individual development or evolutionary development looks smooth or not depends on the time scale one uses.

III. Self-organization, and nonlinear progressions and patterns are quite important in conceptualizing the development of the human mind. Similar patterns may characterize evolution.

 A. Both the mind and behavior patterns emerge during stages in ways that are self-organizing—they develop from the system's own internal feedback systems.

 B. Many key motor, cognitive, and behavioral systems show sudden, nonlinear progressions. After a period of relative stasis, small individual fluctuations can rather quickly stabilize into new forms and patterns.

 C. At a much larger scale, evolution and the development of new species do not occur gradually and linearly but rather through punctuated equilibrium.

IV. Risk and protective factors constitute an important area of studies of the human mind.

 A. A risk factor exists prior to the negative outcome of interest and statistically predicts the outcome's occurrence

 B. Several types of risk factors exist: Fixed risk factors cannot be easily altered: Male verses female status, or temperamental ease verses difficulty. Malleable risk factors are modifiable: parenting styles or schools.

 C. Spurious risk factors appear to predict negative outcomes, but do so only because they are themselves correlated with other, more essential factors.

 D. The premium is discovering causal risk factors. Yet it is quite difficult to understand their nature, as it is practically, and ethically, impossible to do an experiment and randomly assign some youth to conditions of abuse and others to non-abusive environments.

 E. To predict outcomes optimally, we must examine multiple risk factors. The presence of any 1 risk factor does not greatly increase the likelihood of negative outcomes, but 2 risk factors produce a much higher likelihood—and so on.

V. Not everyone exposed to 1 or more risk factor inevitably shows poor outcome. So, the question becomes how to understand those who defy the odds.

  A. Resilience is the set of processes that can yield better-than-expected outcome, in the presence of risk factors.

  B. The search is underway to define protective factors, those qualities or experiences that, under conditions of high risk, produce competence and strength.

Suggested Reading:

Beauchaine and Hinshaw, *Child Psychopathology.*

Werner, *Overcoming the Odds.*

Questions to Consider:

1. Discuss some of the parallels between individual development and evolution, with respect to biology and context, continuities and discontinuities, and the like.

2. What are the contextual factors, including risk and protective factors, that shaped your own and your family's development?

3. Should policies designed to reduce suffering from trauma, poverty, and/or mental illness focus more on reducing risk factors or promoting protective factors?

Lecture Thirteen—Transcript
Parallels between Development and Evolution

In our last lecture, we covered differences between the 2 sexes, and how sex and gender are linked to the brain and mind, evolution and socialization. Today we focus on a big attempt to bring together several key points about individual development, and to show how parallel these principles are in application to evolution and natural selection. We'll begin by taking a broad view of reciprocal determinism, then move on to consider several key concepts: continuity versus discontinuity; self-organization; and resilience. For each of these, we'll be looking foremost at individual development, but we'll be considering strongly parallels at the evolutionary level. This should pull together a lot of what we've discussed so far into a kind of grand integration, so let's begin our journey.

The key point to begin this lecture concerns reciprocal determinism: In shaping the mind, and especially individual differences between minds, environment and biology operate in tandem. What does "in tandem" mean? First, it's completely clear that genes—shaped by evolution—and experience must work hand in hand to create the organism. This isn't some kind of radical statement, it's simply a truism. As we learned in high school in biology, the phenotype—that is, the set of observable characteristics of any organism—is the genotype, as shaped by experience and context. More controversial, though, is the role of genes and biology on the one hand, versus experience and context on the other, in molding differences between individuals. That's the topic of our next lecture, which deals explicitly with behavior genetics and heritability.

How do biology and experience work together at the level of a given individual, or at the level of an entire species? On both of these levels, they do so by repeated patterns of reciprocal and transactional influence, a point first raised in Lecture Nine with respect to child influences and parenting influences working together. How does this reciprocal determinism work? In the case of individual development, one variable (let's say a gene) has an effect on a downstream process—it codes for a protein, maybe helping to sculpt a brain, which creates behavior—but that behavior, in turn, influences the genetic tendency in the future in a kind of relentless spiral.

Let's go straight to behavior, and examine temperament again, which we discussed in Lecture Eight. Shy temperament in the child tends to "pull" the parent to protect him or her; but this protectiveness exacerbates the initial shyness, driving the parent to be even more protective. Who would want to make that poor little thing upset? A positive feedback loop is clearly occurring now. Or, let's take an active, dysregulated temperament in another child: On average, caregivers will be frustrated; and they, in fact, may share genes with the child that further leads them to be impulsive and angrier than the norm in another spiral. The child's tendencies pull the caregiver to fight fire with fire; but this response only makes the child's frustration and dysregulation stronger, another example of a positive feedback loop.

In recent research on reading skill and reading disability, there's another parallel, and it really has profound implications: Some youth, maybe 10% of the population, have genetically mediated problems in the preschool years in learning to form rhymes, or to make those initial correspondences between written symbols and sounds; they're at significant risk for dyslexia and reading disability, which are a source of major impairment in our literacy-driven culture. Research has shown that even in first and second grade, and then as we continue on through the elementary school years, children who read well may encounter more words just in their incidental reading in 2 days than a disabled reader may encounter in one full year. This is alarming and quite tragic; and it clearly shows the multiplier effect of an initial set of problems, leading in this case to curtailing the experience of reading, which only compounds the initial problems—because there's no practice in reading—in a very major way.

Here's the link we're looking for: The same kinds of transactional processes characterize evolution and natural selection, but, of course, on a larger scale and a much longer time frame. Specifically, a mutation could induce a behavior change that is adaptive in a certain environment; although, as we've emphasized, most mutations are not adaptive in unchanging environments. The environment "produces" selection pressure favoring survival and reproduction for those individuals with the mutation, which has produced slightly new structures, or new behavior patterns, rendering the organism more fit. Within a few generations, that particular, mutated gene becomes less rare. Remember, again, Darwin's moths: The gene producing black individual moths were no longer mutants but rather adaptive phenotypes, as the tree trunks and branches became increasingly dark.

The allele frequency can rise from very small fractions—very rare mutations at the beginning phase—to quite substantial frequencies in even 15 or 20 generations. They can become very widespread over a hundred or 2 generations because of the transactional, positive feedback loop that has come to exist in this changing environment. In many cases, a situation comes up where a substantial proportion of the population has one allele, and another substantial proportion carries a different form of the allele; meaning that evolution has clearly favored diversity within that species. It must have been beneficial overall for some individuals to have one kind of physical characteristic or behavioral style, and others to have a different style. This really seems to be the case with regard to human behavior: We have evidence now that 2 or more alleles of genes that code for such neural entities as the serotonin transporter or the dopamine type 4 receptor—which is important for attention and impulse control—are at relatively high proportions in the human species. At the level of behavior, some individuals are shyer and more inhibited, and others bolder; both have been able to prosper. This is a key point to which we'll return.

Taking this reciprocal and transactional argument even a bit further, in some cases the new traits or new behaviors of the organism loop back to transform the environment, producing even stronger selection pressure; so it's a magnified feedback loop. Let's recall again that example of the giraffe's long neck: Mutations producing slight increases in neck size were favored via selection pressure; those giraffes could reach the taller branches. But as this process ensued, taller-necked giraffes would eat more leaves, changing the environment for the trees; the trees, in turn, would undergo selection pressure to grow even taller. This is co-evolution across species in this example.

Here's the overall point: In the development of each individual, and in the development of any species, biology—of course, including the genes in each of our cells—literally interacts with the environment and with context to produce change. In terms of our minds, we can now see how mutations related to the neural density at the cortex, to increased tendencies for myelination, or enlargement of certain regions related to the processing of sounds—speech sounds in particular—would have been favored. Even very small changes initially could have produced just enough enhanced survival and reproduction to make a difference. But over time, these could produce a different level of culture in humans, now verbal and linguistic; and these would favor, in turn, more adaptations, leading initially and then eventually to these increased skills. All of these concepts include some of our best guesses regarding the interaction of our 2 core themes in the course: the individual development of our minds, and evolutionary forces that molded our minds as an entire species.

This parallelism I'm discussing doesn't mean that ontogeny recapitulates phylogeny, the way it was proposed back in the 19th century. Again, human embryos and fetuses don't go through each phase of phylogenetic development, mimicking all species in evolutionary time. What is parallel, rather, is that biology and context matter in reciprocal ways for the development of the individual and the development of species.

Let's take up a key question, related both to individual development and evolution by natural selection: Do these processes of development and change occur smoothly and continuously; or, rather, do they occur in stages, by "jumps and starts," discontinuously? This is a tiny bit of a trick question; if we graph development, it might look smooth or it might not depending on the time scale and the unit of measurement. Let's take an example: How does any individual grow across first 18 years of life? If we plot actual height, year by year, it looks relatively smooth and continuous across time; there's a rise in adolescence, of course, but the curve is still pretty smooth. But what if we, instead, plot the change in height each year, not just the absolute height? This display is not continuous at all; it shows in some phases—the first 2 years of life, early adolescence—big spurts, but hardly any changes in others. What looked fairly smooth in the first graph doesn't look that way at all now. Why is the first graph smooth? Because the "base," or the denominator, is one's overall height; so any change is relatively small compared to that number of inches or centimeters in the denominator. But the second graph is simply change; it's quite bumpy, because some years are marked by considerable growth, and others are marked by very little. There's no big denominator to smooth things out.

The same thing could be true of the evolution of species, again depending on the time units of the graph we create. Evolution is "conservative"—literally, features tend to be conserved across generations—given that radical mutations would, in all likelihood, not be successful. But consider this: If the environment is changing quite rapidly or radically—think of the tree bark again back in 19th-century England—one single mutation could actually lead to fairly sudden change. Again, whether growth is continuous or discontinuous depends largely on the scale of measurement.

Let's go beyond height to look at some examples more closely related to the mind. Let's look at spoken language: It shows in most children a big spurt around 18 months of age; of course, it could be earlier, sometimes a bit or even much later. Remember multiple levels of analysis: This is a prime era for synaptogenesis and pruning. It could well be that any specific genes related to brain regions responsible for language come online—they get switched on—at such periods.

Thinking of cognitive development, let's recall Piaget's stages back from Lectures 8 and 9. Piaget said they are just that: They are stages; they are qualitative, discontinuous leaps in mental function. After a long period, even years, of relative stasis, biological maturation and the child's specific interactions with the world lead to a relatively sudden burst of understanding; for example, in concrete operations, that the volume of a fluid depends on both the width and height of the container. Concrete operations in this view encompass a new stage, a leap, in cognitive development. This is somewhat controversial: Some research tells us that children may achieve development of some Piagetian stages earlier than Piaget thought and even more gradually, and that explicit teaching might actually help a child develop concrete operations before the normal maturational unfolding and that leap would normally occur.

Here's something quite interesting: At the times when marked discontinuities do occur in individual development, this is often a signal of important underlying shifts in our brains and minds. It could be an indicator of changes at lower or higher "levels of analysis"; so maybe a gene has suddenly been expressed with downstream effects. Thinking of adolescents, maybe wider exposure to contexts outside the family is occurring right near the time of maximum hormonal bursts, so that a qualitative change in cognitive processes could ensue. At these times, development is quite likely to be discontinuous or nonlinear. Sometimes we call these periods "phase shifts," and this is borrowed from chemistry and physics. Think of water as it freezes into ice; very suddenly, at 32 degrees Fahrenheit, the molecules realign, although they have really not done so at each degree of cooling before we got down to 32 degrees Fahrenheit.

In other words, systems can undergo radical shifts quite suddenly; a new structure, a new set of behaviors can emerge with maybe just a small additional change in conditions (in the example we just gave, temperature). These changes we define as nonlinear; they don't follow any kind of straight path. Developmentalists consider a child's learning to walk as a prime example: After a lot of false starts, many steps cruising with hands on the sofa for support, suddenly, the first few unassisted steps emerge. The average age for this is right around 12 months, but there is, of course, great variation across children. Here's a memory from our first-born son, many years ago when he was just about 4 ½ months of age: I can remember vividly that he'd been trying for some weeks, lying on the living room rug, to roll over. One night in April—I can recall it as if it was yesterday—he succeeded, made his first roll over, and with a big smile of obvious delight, he rolled over again and again, about 30 times in a row.

Presaging our discussions in later lectures of what can happen when the mind "goes wrong," mental illness develops: It could be that what are apparently tiny issues or problems, just before the time that rapid change ensues, get magnified. Think of adolescence, the time period in which many serious mental disorders emerge in full form. Even a small crack in the foundation might become enormous—Earthquake-like, to take a physical example—when adolescence ensues.

Phase shifts within individual development are related to an important concept we call "self-organization"; this is applicable to both individual development and natural selection. What do we mean? The mind and many behavior patterns emerge from early phases and stages in ways that are self-organizing; that is, they develop from the system's own internal feedback systems. Once initial conditions have been set in motion, the process tends to unfold of its own accord. When this process occurs, we can't really explain some of the higher-order effects on the basis of the lower-order components; our minds think, but components of our minds—neurons—don't think on their own. Something emergent happens when neurons come together in the incredibly complex ways that they do. As just discussed, many motor, cognitive, and behavioral systems reveal fairly sudden, nonlinear progressions. After a period of relative stasis, small individual fluctuations, predicted by biological maturity, and/or environmental "press" and opportunity, can rather quickly stabilize into new forms and patterns.

Here's the parallel: At a much larger time scale—that of evolution—development of new species does not occur gradually and linearly, but rather through a process called "punctuated equilibrium." Species tend to be stable, once formed, if the ecosystem stays relatively constant. But climate changes, or other ecosystem changes, might rather quickly occur in geological time. Consider the state of the Earth after a huge asteroid—of course, it was a meteorite once it hit the Earth—plunged into what is now the Yucatan Peninsula 65 million years ago. It created a kind of huge, long-lasting, catastrophic winter that helped lead to the extinction of dinosaurs, and indeed over half of the other species on Earth. After millions of years of rather gradual, linear changes in evolution—prompted by mutations, some of which became naturally selected—this kind of sudden environmental change prompted non-linear, self-organizing changes in speciation. There have actually been several other radical changes in speciation on Earth across evolution, some even more radical than this event.

Like individual development, evolution comes in spurts, rather than appearing in smooth, linear, continuous form. Genes and environments self-organize into species in ways that are parallel to individual nonlinear change; and remember from Lecture Seven, microevolution, subtle but essential changes in gene expression related to language areas of the brain and other key elements of the human mind. When we think of this, an issue gets re-raised: Maybe the skills and strengths of our minds have been conserved from our primate ancestors; language, for example—mythic skills—emanate from gesture and mimetic skills in other primates. But the newer consideration is this: Maybe humans truly differ in a discontinuous way from our ancestors. Maybe there are more than just quantitative differences of degree—we have more of the skill, other primates have less—but truly qualitative differences, discontinuous ones: We have unique skills that they didn't have.

Recent microevolution and cognitive science, taking a hard look at the evidence, has come to the view that many human skills may, in fact, be more qualitatively different from those of our closest relatives than had been thought. Some chimps can learn sign languages, but none has truly emerged with a unique grammar, the way that almost every single human 2- and 3-year-old does. This is a big topic and a fascinating one; it's really gone back and forth throughout the history of evolutionary science and the history of philosophy.

Spirit-based and humanistic views of the mind, back from Lecture One, have almost uniformly held that humans are unique, separate from other species; but then evolutionary subsequently posited more gradual, progressive change. But remember the article I quoted back in Lecture One by Penn, Holyoak, and Povinelli; it was entitled "Darwin's Mistake," and talked about all those uniquely human skills. The contention of this article and other recent science is that Darwin, and other evolutionists, have actually underestimated some key, qualitative differences in human minds as opposed to those of other species. Grammatical language, the ability to create narratives, time travel, and empathy are just 4 examples of skills that, although they emerged from other species, are qualitatively uniquely different in humans. The debate rages still; and we'll get back to it in our last lecture when we consider the future of the human mind.

Let's continue with individual development, and now examine a concept called "resilience." The basic idea is that there are 2 important kinds of processes for developing positive resilience in the human mind; we'll call them "risk factors" and "protective factors." A "risk factor" is a force, a condition, an individual trait that exists prior to some outcome we're interested in—usually a negative outcome—and it statistically predicts that the outcome will occur later on. What's a risk factor for aggression and delinquency in adolescents? Being male; having an XY chromosome pattern on 23. One is male before becoming delinquent, and being male predicts higher rates of delinquency than does being female. This is an example of what we call a "fixed risk factor"; we cannot easily alter being male or female. Malleable risk factors, on the other hand, could be modifiable: parenting styles, types of schools.

There's another kind of risk factor we call "spurious." These are ones that appear to predict negative outcomes, but they actually do so only because they themselves are associated with other, more essential factors. Here's an important example: It's been known for some time that minority racial status predicts aggression and delinquency, but actually, its effects are spurious. When we control for the fact that African-American youth are on average poorer than majority youth, it's the poverty, not the racial status, that's actually the stronger predictor.

What's the Holy Grail here? Discovering "causal" risk factors; these are the ones that are not only malleable but also the true reasons for increases in the outcomes of interest. But it's hard to know what is a causal risk factor; because of practicalities and ethics it's very hard to do a random assignment experiment, and, for example, delegate some youth to conditions of abuse and others to non-abusive environments, or to make some individuals be born male and others female.

Our optimal predictions come when we look at multiple risk factors; risk factors working together. Often, any single risk factor doesn't greatly increase the likelihood of a bad outcome; but 2 together often produce a much higher chance, 3 even more, and so on. Here's an example: Both early biological risk (defined as prenatal problems and birth complications) and early psychosocial rejection in the first year of life (attempted abortion, placement of an infant outside the home during the first year) are implicated here. Neither one of those is a very predictive risk factor of antisocial behavior by early adulthood; but the combination is a pretty potent one. It takes both the biological and early psychosocial rejection combined to enhance the risk.

There are many risk factors for problems in our mental well-being. This could span traumatic experiences, abuse, poverty, having a parent with a mental illness, being born with a very difficult temperament, living in a violent neighborhood; these are just a couple of examples. But here's the essential point: Not everyone exposed to one or more risk factors inevitably shows poor outcome. How do we understand those who "defy the odds?" "Resilience" is the term signifying the set of processes that can yield better-than-expected outcomes, even in the presence of risk factors. If we find this occurring, we have to search for protective factors; those qualities of the individual or those life experiences that, under conditions of high risk, produce competence, strength, and resilience.

Early research in this area back in the 1960s focused on the term "invulnerable" children. In this view, there are a few children, despite high risk, who just simply thrive. Resiliency was thought to be an "all or none" characteristic; protective factors were those inside the individual's skin. But we now know that it's really not that simple at all: Resilience is not all or none; a child at risk because of poverty, family mental illness, or abuse or neglect may be doing well academically but suffering badly socially. We have to consider this: Resilience is more than doing well in just one domain. We wouldn't want to call an adolescent girl with a serious eating disorder like anorexia "resilient" simply because she's doing well in school—actually, this could be a sign of the perfectionism that many such girls may display—at the same time she could be literally starving herself. We have to consider several factors.

How do we label or consider protective factors? Some do exist within the individual: high intelligence can be protective; a sense of humor; an orientation toward the future. More protective factors emerge from key life relationships: family discipline styles; support outside the home. Still other protective factors exist at the level of the neighborhood or community: safe neighborhoods, less violent ones; perhaps smaller class size; etc. Supportive relationships may be the crucial protective factor when we consider all research on this topic. For youth without a very good home life, some kind of mentor/advocate outside the home appears to be crucial in bolstering the chances of combating high risk; it promotes resilience. Some schools and some teachers appear to be quite good at helping children with high risk for behavioral or emotional problems to fare well socially and academically. Teachers who value multiple areas of strength rather than a single, rigid standard of academic success may be particularly good at promoting academic and social competence.

My colleague Ann Masten, Professor at the University of Minnesota, is a world expert on resilience, and she contends that the processes that foster resilient functioning are not some kinds of strange, remarkable esoteric factors but she calls them "ordinary magic"; everyday processes—good parenting, supportive relationships, safety in neighborhoods, the building of confidence and competence, skill teaching—that all of us can foster.

Here's an intriguing fact: Genes themselves could be protective factors. In an interesting study from Britain, high-risk identical twins were more likely to both be resilient in the face of adversity and poverty than were high-risk fraternal twins; so something about the shared genes promoted resilience. There's not a resilience gene per se; there may be many genes combining and shaping our approach to the world that help us to be protected.

The perspective of resilience really forces us to consider strengths and competencies. Much of clinical psychology and psychiatry necessarily focuses on pathology, difficult outcomes, and mental illness. This is not totally inappropriate—we go to the mechanic when our cars aren't working; we go to the therapist when behaviors, emotional patterns, or relationships aren't working right—but unlike cars, people are far more complex; they're reciprocal and transactional. It may really help to relieve symptoms by focusing on competence and strength, and not just weakness. Perhaps the way to health of our minds is truly to focus on developing competencies, not just eliminating symptoms.

We've covered a lot of ground today; the bottom line is this: Human behavior, human emotion, and the human mind are complex products of biology and experience, operating reciprocally, transactionally, and often in non-linear form. Similarly, evolution operates via a parallel set of processes, although on a far longer time scale. People, like other complex systems, self-organize, showing emergent properties not reducible to the underlying components that seem to have created them. The same is true for species and other processes related to natural selection.

Finally, the study of risk factors, protective factors, and resilience tells us about the importance of strength and competence, not just problems and pathology. A positive orientation to the development of the individual human mind is not just being "Pollyannaish," but may be the key to understanding both pathology and optimal development. The origins of the human mind are not simple; related to individual development and species development, complex reciprocal and transactional processes are at work. Would we expect it any differently, given our 120 billion or more neurons, their almost unfathomable interconnections, our penchant for plasticity, and the richness of our physical and social environments?

It may well be that to promote survival and thriving, evolution has provided for some still-mysterious mechanisms that promote strength in the face of adversity, which we can attempt to find and use in changing individual development. Resilient functioning is, indeed, a core feature of the human mind.

Lecture Fourteen
Myths and Realities of Heritability

Scope:

With the decoding of the human genome in the beginning of the 21st century, there has been a major resurgence of interest in genes, particularly with respect to their influences in shaping behavior. This lecture emphasizes behavioral genetics, including the use of twin and adoption studies to infer heritability. A number of misconceptions related to heritability are considered, including the notions that high heritability signals the workings of a single gene, that heritability negates any role of the environment in influencing minds and behaviors, and that heritability is destiny.

Outline

I. Following a period of relative neglect throughout much of the 20th century, when environmental influences on behavior and the human mind were dominant, there has been a major resurgence of interest in genes and their influence on behavior across the past several decades.

   A. The decoding of the human genome at the beginning of the 21st century set the stage for a new area of work on genetic influences.

   B. In this lecture and the next, we will see that it is a combination of genes and environments that always make the key difference. And, epigenetic forces—factors that influence gene expression but are not a direct part of genetic material—are essential to consider.

II. The concept of heritability is quite important for establishing the effects of genes on behavior and the mind—yet it can be quite misunderstood.

   A. Many believe that a particular behavior, trait, or emotio, is the product genes versus environments.

   B. But any common trait is actually the full product of both genes and environments; we can't separate out the influences.

C. It does make sense, however, to talk about differences across people—and the extent to which such difference are attributable more to genetic influences or environmental influences.

III. Heritability is a statistic that gives the percentage, from 0 to 100, as to whether difference between people are attributable to genes; all environmental influences are considered 0% heritable, where as 100% signifies all genetic.

    A. How do we infer heritability? The typical methods are family or pedigree studies, comparing risk across various relatives; and twin studies, comparing identical twins to fraternal twins, Both are confounded, in part, by similar environments in close relatives.

    B. If there is greater concordance in identical twin pairs than fraternal twin pairs, heritability can be assumed. Identical twins reared apart from infancy provide an even better test.

    C. Adoption studies are also used, with the aim of determining whether biological versus adoptive relatives are more similar in a given trait, behavior, or condition.

IV. A number of misconceptions are found in relation to the concept of heritability.

    A. Many believe that a high heritability reflects the effects of a single gene on the behavior or trait in question.

    B. Heritability refers to the relative influence of genes, rather than environments, on individual differences in a trait or behavior in a given population at a given point in time. It does not pertain to the percentage of any individual's liability for the trait or behavior.

    C. Most people believe that heritability implies stability of the trait in question across generations. But, in fact, the overall levels of a highly heritable trait or behavior, over time, may be dependent on environments, not genes.

    D. Many contend that genes tell us everything about behaviors and traits with moderate to high heritability. It is mistaken to think that heritable traits and conditions are completely refractory to environmental input, in order to alter the course of the condition for individuals.

V. The overall point is that there is great malleability in human behavior, even though genes may set a number of preconditions.

Suggested Reading:

Plomin, DeFries, McClearn, and McGuffin, *Behavioral Genetics*.

Rutter, *Genes and Behavior*.

Questions to Consider:

1. Why is a trait or condition that is moderately or strongly heritable still able to be influenced by the environment in terms of its long-term outcomes?

2. What are some of the key factors that may be related to the recent decreases in aggression and antisocial behavior among boys, as well as the recent increases in such behavior patterns in girls?

Lecture Fourteen—Transcript
Myths and Realities of Heritability

Given the plasticity of our minds, which we've, of course, emphasized a lot in our past lectures, how is it that genes and environments work together in shaping our emotions, behaviors, and minds overall? Genes are not a complete blueprint; but our minds are not blank slates, either. The material today should challenge some things that you've learned in the past; it clearly reflects a lot of exciting new science.

To say that we're in the era of genetics and genomics in human sciences is really an understatement. Genes, and evolution in general, were quite neglected for the first decades of the 20th century, in psychology and the behavioral sciences overall. Environmental influences on behavior and the human mind were the dominant influences. Scientists doubted that there was really such a thing as temperament, reflecting early behavioral effects of genetic predispositions; or if it existed, temperament was thought to be really pretty unimportant. Psychodynamic and social learning principles were what everyone in the field talked about and learned. In terms of any behavior, the stereotype was, "My parents made me do it." The effects of culture and of learning were believed to be the dominant influences on the human mind. Anthropologists emphasized how different the different cultures on our planet really are, and how cultures, rather than any underlying biology, were the predominant influence on development and minds.

Many in the field really didn't want to get into the kinds of noxious Social Darwinism that had ruled for much of the late 19th and early 20th centuries, which blamed the underclass of society for their ineffective or even deviant genes. Political views undoubtedly played a role here: Why limit human potential by discussing biological programs or genetic limits on behavior? Why even consider that males and females might have biologically-determined differences; wouldn't that be inherently sexist? But in the last 40 years or so, there has been a major resurgence of interest in genes and their influence on behavior.

Every time we discuss genes, by definition we're bringing in the concept of natural selection, because it is adaptive genes, in the context of a particular environment, that are passed on to the next generation in this concept of reproduction of the fittest. Evolution works directly through genes; natural selection promotes genes, producing organisms with the strongest chances of reproducing in a real positive feedback loop.

A major new surge of interest came about at the beginning of the 21st century, when both federal investigators and a private firm led by Craig Ventner finally put forward the announcement that their joint venture had decoded the human genome. We now know the composition of all 3 billion base pairs of nucleotides inside the nucleus inside each of our trillions of cells. This mass of DNA is divided, in humans, into about 20,000 genes. In classic theory, each gene codes for a certain set of amino acids, making proteins, the building blocks of life. But from Lecture Seven, recall that there are certain genes that don't just code for a certain protein; some genes are master genes, or toolkit genes, having the effect of producing RNA that regulates multiple other genes at key times in development. The 99% of our DNA that is not located on any particular gene is not any longer considered just "mystery DNA" or "junk DNA," it may actually help regulate the DNA that is located on genes.

In recent decades, rather than what was said in the past—"My culture made me do it," or "My parents made me do it"; or, maybe in Freudian terms, "My id made me do it"—the claim most recently has been that, "My genes made me do it." But this is simplistic, reductionistic, and misguided; as one-sided as the view that parents and culture were the sole determinants of all individual differences. There are no specific genes for any specific form of behavior. Genes make RNA and proteins; those proteins, in turn, develop into larger structures and whole organs and brains, eventually organisms. The linkage between genes and behaviors is complex, bringing to mind the multiple levels of analysis introduced back in Lecture One.

We're going to focus now on the ways in which genes work to shape brain structures and the functions of our mind, but we must consider also what are called "epigenetic" forces and factors, those biological and even experiential forces outside of DNA, per se, which are essential to how genes function. For some time, well before we even knew that genes were composed of DNA, scientists knew through studies of twins and adoptees about the overall effects of many genes on traits, behaviors, and conditions of interest. This is the field called "behavioral genetics." This is a crucial area, full of misunderstanding, so pay some close attention.

The key concept from behavioral genetics is heritability; how much genes, not environments, cause individual differences in a trait or condition. Let's first deal with a key misunderstanding: Some of us believe that a particular behavior, trait, emotion, or condition is the product of either genes or environments, with some relative percentage given to each; but that's just not right. Any what we call "common trait"—a trait that all humans share to some extent—is the full product of both genes and environments, as we discussed last time; we can't separate out those influences. My height, your irritability, her optimism, or his aggression are 100% a product of genes and 100% a product of environments; but you really can't break it down any further. But what does make sense is to talk about differences across people; the extent to which such differences are attributable, more to either genetic influences or environmental influences.

Let's stay with this example of how tall or short each of us is: Human height is distributed almost perfectly on a bell curve: a few extremely tall individuals, a few extremely short individuals, and most falling in between the extremes; the great majority bunch near the mean or average. Here's the key question: Are the differences in height across the population—technically, the variability or variance in height—related more to genetic differences across people or to differences in the environments in which they were raised? Heritability is the statistic—it's a percentage, from 0–100%—telling us whether differences between people are attributable to genes (100% means "all genetic") or to environments (0% means "not genetic," all environmental). Heritability, again, doesn't mean that my height or your height is a certain degree or percentage genetic; it refers to the genetic versus environmental reasons for why you and I differ in our heights. For example, a different example is the tendency to baldness—or, maybe in my case, gray hair—heritable or more environmental across people?

How do we get estimates of heritability? The first method is called "family" or "pedigree" studies. Here's the key premise: If I'm related to you, I share genes with you; the more closely related I am to you, the more genes I tend to share with you; and therefore, the more likely I should be to share a similar trait, behavior, or condition with you. What's the catch? The more related I am to you, the more likely I am also to share an environment with you; I may even live with you if you're my parent or my sibling. Family studies can provide only circumstantial evidence for heritability; it would obviously be best to rule out environmental similarities, too, which we'll discuss.

Let's take a key example: What about the risk for developing the devastating mental disorder called schizophrenia, which we'll discuss more in Lecture Seventeen. How does the risk relate to genetic relatedness to someone with this disorder? If I'm unrelated to someone with schizophrenia, what are my chances of developing it? About 1%; that's the prevalence of the condition in the population. If I'm a distant relative, however—a biological relative—my chances climb over 1%; and if I'm a close relative, my chances grow much higher. In fact, if both of my parents have schizophrenia, the chances are about 50/50 that I will develop this condition myself. This evidence is consistent with the contention that schizophrenia is heritable; but, of course, it's not definitive, because we haven't completely separated genes from environments.

The logical extension of family studies is twin studies. Here, we compare identical twins (called monozygotic twins, from the same fertilized egg) who share all of their genes, to fraternal (or dizygotic twins, who, just like any siblings, share about half of their genes). What we do is calculate the "concordance" between twin pairs; that's the proportion of twins who both have the trait (both are tall, both are aggressive, both have schizophrenia). The greater the concordance in identical twin pairs than in fraternal twin pairs, the higher the heritability. There's a specific formula here: Very roughly, heritability is equivalent to 2 times the difference in the identical versus fraternal twin concordance rates. If the monozygotic or identical rate is .5 concordance and the dizygotic or fraternal rate is .2, heritability very roughly, would be about 2 times the difference, .3, or .6; 60%. The assumption here is that identical twins, of course, are twice as genetically related as fraternal twins, but the environments are the same. Yet isn't it the case that identical twins are actually treated more similarly? Yes, perhaps so; but the reason may well be because very similarity in appearance drives more similar treatment from parents and teachers. Again, remember reciprocal causation—parent behavior causes child behavior, and child's characteristics drives parent responses—are pertinent here.

©2010 The Teaching Company.

What would be a really ideal test? What about identical twins that were separated at birth, never met, and were reared in completely different environments. Let's get technical: even they shared the same prenatal environment; still, however, this is a better way to separate genes from postnatal environment. What do such studies show? Identical twins raised apart are pretty likely to have similarities, not only in terms of physical characteristics—which we might expect—but also in terms of behaviors and personality traits, and even liability for mental illness. This gets to be pretty strong evidence for heritability. But the sheer numbers of identical twins reared apart from birth are quite small, and this is problematic for getting good estimates of the heritability of a condition like schizophrenia, which is pretty rare.

What's the third method, after family and twin studies? These are adoption studies. The goal here is to see whether a biological relative versus an adoptive relatives is more similar in a given trait, behavior, or condition. If I share half of my genes with you, because you are my parent, but I've never met you or interacted with you because I was adopted away at birth, am I more like you than I am my adoptive parents, with whom I don't share any genes, but who raised me? One problem with this method is that when infants are adopted, they are somewhat likely to go into homes that are somewhat similar in terms of economic and educational level to those of their biological parents. If you're getting my point here, adoption studies may under-represent the importance of environments, because there's not the full range of environments under which adoptees may go. Still, adoption studies show that a big part of the risk for height, personality traits, and even mental disorders like schizophrenia is attributable to genetic rather than environmental relatedness.

Let's go for a few examples here. How heritable is height? What I'm asking here again is: How much are the differences across people in height related genes or environment? The answer is that height is about 90% heritable; almost all of the differences across people in terms of their height are related to their genes, not their environments. What about other instances that might be related more to the mind? Let's take religious affiliations: Which particular religion may be your choice? The very low heritability here means that which religion you or I choose is related almost exclusively to our families of origin or our cultural beliefs. On the other hand, differences between people in the likelihood of having strong spiritual beliefs overall, regardless of the type, has a pretty strong heritability. The content of religious beliefs is not very heritable at all, but the presence of such beliefs is much more so.

Back to some of our past lectures: What about temperamental or personality? The short answer here is that activity level, aggression, and effortful control during the earliest years of life are mildly, to modestly, to sometimes moderately heritable. But as we get older, adult personality traits like conscientiousness (diligence), neuroticism (our ability to see the negative in most situations), and extraversion (one's love of parties versus spending time alone) all have heritabilities of 50%, or even slightly more; there's a little bit of variability around that, but on average half. Genes have more to do with behaviors and personality traits than we once thought. But let's remember, of course, that there isn't a gene for conscientiousness, or a gene for height; what's inherited is a set of genes, which sum together to yield the template for the trait in question.

There are a number of key misconceptions, even myths, about heritability and what it means. Let's take them up one by one, as they reveal some fascinating concepts and should help us to appreciate all the more reciprocal and transactional processes in the development of the mind, rather than reductionistic notions of genes or environments operating in isolation. In fact, I think it might not be a bad idea to either scrap the term "heritability" altogether, which too often implies the immutable effects of genes; or at least to pay very close attention to what it really does and does not signify.

Here's the first misconception or myth: As we just discussed, commonly it's believed that high heritability means there's a single gene that's responsible. Again, let's just take height: very high heritability, 90%; but there's no height gene. It may be that there are hundreds, even thousands of our genes, acting together that provide the maximum ceiling on an individual's potential ultimate height. The same is true for the personality traits and behaviors we just discussed: Conscientiousness, negativity and neuroticism, agreeableness, all of the "Big Five" factors, are, again, about 50% heritable; but there's no single gene for any of these personality traits.

We'll discuss a bit later in this course that many forms of mental illness have heritabilities that are way above zero: depression is 30–40% heritable. Bipolar disorder, on the other hand—manic-depressive illness—much higher, around 80%. But there's no single gene for these forms of mental disorder as well. Certain neurological conditions—Huntington's disease, or Duchenne muscular dystrophy—are, in fact, related to single genes. But the most lethal medical conditions—heart disease, cancers, lung conditions—are polygenic, meaning that multiple genes are involved, interacting with one another and with the environment in complex ways; the same is true for mental disorders.

What about the second myth or misconception? It's often thought that if a trait has a high heritability, environments are just unimportant related to the expression of that trait; I mean if heritability is high, it's genes that matter, right? That's all. But we need to be precise in our definition: "Heritability" refers to the relative influence of genes, rather than environments, on individual differences in a trait or behavior in a given population at a given point in time. Different subpopulations of humans with different frequencies of various genes may have actually different heritabilities for the same trait or condition; and if environments change, so can heritabilities. This may sound difficult, or even strange; let's examine it in some detail.

Here's an example that might strike you as counterintuitive initially; if you can understand this, you'll probably be a lot further in getting this topic. Intelligence, measured by IQ tests, has a moderately strong heritability; genes have a lot to say about differences between people in their IQ test scores. Depending on the test and the sample, heritability is around 60%. We know this from twin and adoption studies. I must add: A big question is whether IQ tests really measure "intelligence"; this is hotly debated. Some experts conceptualize intelligence as constituting multiple functions, some of which are well beyond the scope of most standard IQ tests.

But we'll stop that digression for now about the ultimate nature of intelligence. Consider this point: What if we could somehow magically tomorrow equalize all schools and all home environments in order to promote higher intelligence in children. What would be the implications for IQ and its heritability? If we could do that, what would the heritability of IQ be? It would become 100%. Why? Because now, all of the variability in IQ would be related to genes, not environments. Paradoxically, then, trying to ensure equality of opportunity would only accentuate genetically based differences in IQ scores. Take the parallel, a little harder to conceptualize: what if we could alter those genes responsible for IQ in order to help boost IQs of children with somewhat lower ones. This is a bit of a stretch; but to the extent that this could be possible, the heritabilities for IQ would go down, not up, because environments would now be the main difference if genetic contributions and contributors were equalized. How would we say this in scientific language? Heritability is context-dependent: As situations change—as genes mutate—or as environments become more or less important or variable, heritability can change, too.

Let's proceed to our third myth: If heritability is high, a trait or a condition is fixed, locked in by genes, and it stays that way across generations. Let's go back to height again: Height is 90% heritable, as we've discussed; but our entire population in the U.S. is around 3 inches taller than our grandparents and great grandparents were a century ago. The reason is not that height-related genes have quickly mutated across 3 or 4 generations; it would take far longer for such mutations to gain a selective advantage and alter height. What is the reason? It's most likely because of changes in nutrition across the last century: higher fat content, more protein, maybe more hormones in beef, etc. Even for very heritable conditions, changes in the environment or context can raise or lower the level of the entire trait across the whole population. Heritability refers to the relative influence of genes, not environments, at a given time and in a given population; but it doesn't tell us anything about how environments may alter the overall trait across the time and across the whole population.

We discussed in back Lecture Ten puberty and menarche: They are under genetic control, but the age of onset is dropping; over 2 years in the last century, not, again, because of genetic factors but because of environment and nutrition. Fat content in food, higher fat proportion in girls and some boys may have driven earlier puberty.

Certain environments may change the expression of genes, literally switching them on or off without actually altering their DNA inside our chromosomes per se. Genes may or may not be activated for reasons lying outside the gene itself. These are what we call "epigenetic" forces or factors; these are forces acting on our genes, but they're outside DNA per se. What about a behavioral example? Lots of research has shown that boys' rates of violence in the U.S. went up pretty steadily from roughly 1920 until about 1995. Poverty, larger inner cities, modeling of violence, media effects; all of these and many more were offered as explanations. But these are social and cultural factors, not genetic changes per se; violence has moderate heritability, but we wouldn't find an increase in boys over all because of changes in genes within a few decades. But at the same time, since about 1995, boys' rates of aggression and violence have gone down fairly steadily, but girls' rates have gone up by over a third. It must be cultural and social forces, not quick genetic changes in girls that were the culprit leading to increases in violence in a 15-year period.

Final example: IQ scores tend to go up about 3 points every decade (of course, we keep re-norming the test so the mean or average is still 100). IQ is quite heritable; about 60% or more, as we just discussed. Again, quick rises in IQ scores across the population can't be related to gene mutations in a decade or 2 or 3. There's a lot of speculation about what could be driving the increase in intelligence: stimulating preschool environments; maybe a more abstract culture in general, changing the ways that all of us respond to conceptual, abstract questions related to general intelligence.

Myth number 4: Many contend that the effects of genes are really the same for everybody across the whole population. It's just not true; let's take another example related to IQ: Erik Turkheimer, a colleague and psychologist at the University of Virginia, showed that the heritability of IQ depends greatly on one's social class. In other words, IQ is quite heritable for upper-class and upper-middle-class children, but it's far lower for poor children. Why would this be? It's similar to the point just made about variability in environments: There are much wider differences in the rearing and school environments for our most disenfranchised youth, so the relative impact of genes is less because environments tend to matter more. This is really intriguing notion, isn't it? Heritability doesn't stay constant as environments change.

Finally, myth number 5: It's often assumed that heritability implies destiny, and that high heritability for a behavioral or developmental problem implies that the only hope would be to alter genes. We're going to take the example of PKU, phenylketonuria; this is a recessive, genetic disease that is 100% heritable. If you inherit 2 copies of the recessive allele, you get it; heritability is everything, genes are everything here. If you have this disorder, you cannot properly metabolize phenylalanine. Levels therefore build to toxic levels in the brain, and the usual result is moderate to severe mental retardation.

This is a 100% heritable condition; how do we treat PKU? We can't do gene therapy yet, it isn't viable; but what we can do is restrict the intake of certain foods that contain phenylalanine and other chemicals. Certain food labels, even on Diet Coke cans, show that PKU may be triggered by the phenylalanine in the substance. What if we can restrict the diet so that there's no phenylalanine ingested? PKU babies grow with normal IQ scores.

It's a big mistake to think that heritable traits and conditions are totally unresponsive or refractory to environmental input in altering the course of this condition for given individuals. We're going to hear more about this in the case of highly heritable mental and behavioral disorders like ADHD, bipolar disorder, and autism later in the course. Genes matter, but we can treat them through environmental means.

What's our overall point? There is great malleability in human behavior, even though genes may set a number of preconditions. Genes are fixed when we're born; but they're activated by master genes and by what we call "epigenetic" factors and forces, biological and even experiential variables that can switch them on or off. The brain in particular is highly plastic, as we've emphasized throughout the course. Along with genetic instructions, experiences "tell" neurons where and when to make synaptic connections with other neurons; and the human mind has very few absolutely critical periods for development. Recall the devastating examples of the adopted Romanian orphans: Despite in some cases months or even several years of severe deprivation, many cognitive functions could come back, although there were clearly sensitive periods after several years of deprivation.

Today's information should convince you that heritability isn't everything, and that epigenetic influences are essential in shaping the human mind. Our brains and minds are, indeed, malleable. But genes do exert influence; and we're not as completely flexible and malleable as some of our scientific predecessors might have thought, especially early social learning theorists, who posited nearly complete environmental determinism for our blank slate mind.

Next time, we're going to look the precise ways in which genes and environments do work together to create our minds, and the huge individual differences in our emotions, behaviors, and traits. For now, we must realize that biology and experience cannot be separated; that many traits and facets of the mind are more heritable than we would once have imagined; and that without paying careful attention to the facts, myths about heritability abound and we may be in danger of ignoring the huge malleability and its potential in our brains and minds.

Lecture Fifteen
Genes and Environments Together

Scope:

How do genes and contextual factors produce individual differences in behavior? In the additive model of behavioral genetics, the 3 core influences on any traits are genes, shared environments, and non-shared environments—all of which are assumed to be independent of one another. Genes account for at least half of the variation in many traits; intriguingly, non-shared environmental influences are stronger than shared influences, calling into question many classic studies of parenting influences. In gene-environment interaction, certain genotypes are expressed only in certain environments but not others. Thus, genes and environments are interdependent; nature and nurture work together in unexpected ways to yield both strength and pathology.

Outline

I. In the classic additive model of behavioral genetics, there are 3 core influences on behavior and the mind.

   A. Genes: Heritability refers to the effects of genes on individual differences in a behavior or trait.

   B. Shared environment: These influences are those contextual variables that siblings experience together—such as poverty or parental discipline styles that are similar across children.

   C. Non-shared environment: Here, contextual variables differ among siblings. These include parenting practices that diverge across children or the different peer groups experienced by the different children in a family.

   D. The assumption is that all 3 of these influences sum to 100% in terms of their influence on behavioral variability and that they are independent of one another.

II. For most traits that constitute the normal range of human functioning, genes explain a moderate amount of variance, shared environments explain a small portion, but non-shared environments explain an amount comparable to that from genes.

A. This pattern is surprising, as it contradicts the predominant belief that a family's general child-rearing style is extremely influential.

B. The implication is that a range of idiosyncratic, highly individualized experiences determine much more of the human mind than previously believed.

C. An exception to this pattern is the outcome of aggression or antisocial behavior, for which shared environmental factors play a significant role.

III. Considerable research challenges the assumption that these 3 components are actually independent. Genes and environments tend to go together, and certain environments may accentuate the effects of certain genes.

IV. The first important concept is gene-environment correlation—signifying that the genes passed along from parents to children are often associated with the environments in which the children find themselves or create for themselves.

A. The heritability of many behavioral traits increases with age; the implication is that genotypes are accentuated by environments across development.

B. In passive gene-environment correlation, genes that are common to both parents and children influence parenting behaviors.

C. In active gene-environment correlation, the child inherits tendencies from the parents that propel him or her to perform behaviors that accentuate the inherited traits: The child's heritable tendencies influence the selection of environments.

D. In evocative gene-environment correlation, the child's inherited tendencies elicit responses that accentuate existing vulnerabilities.

V. The second important concept is gene-environment interaction. Here, the idea is that environments may well determine whether a gene actually exerts an effect on the mind or on behavior.

A. Several important examples have been discovered by Caspi and colleagues. The first is related to risk for serious depression: A combination the inefficient form of the serotonin transporter gene, plus high levels of negative life events strongly predicted depression by age 26.

B. Unless the 2 factors, genes and environments, have been considered together, it could easily be assumed that the gene had no effect on depression or that life events mattered little.

VI. The essential point is that the common dichotomy of nature versus nurture is outdated and inaccurate. Nature and nurture combine in incredible ways to shape the human mind. Overall, genes and environments are not as separate as one might believe.

Suggested Reading:

There is a host of research on how genes and environments combine in novel ways to shape both positive/adaptive and negative/problematic behavior patterns. The results of such work are found in scientific journals such as *Science, Development and Psychopathology, Archives of General Psychiatry*, and more. Key contributions have been made by Caspi and Moffitt. For the best compilation of theory and research in this area, see Rutter, *Genes and Behavior: Nature-Nurture Interplay Explained.*

Questions to Consider:

1. What is meant by the concept of gene-environment correlation and how does it reveal unique ways that genes and environments work together?

2. What is meant by the concept of gene-environment interaction, and how does it reveal unique ways that genes and environments work together?

Lecture Fifteen—Transcript
Genes and Environments Together

Behavior genetics gives us a kind of 20,000-foot view of genes and environments. Today we move from this broad perspective to a much closer look at the specific ways in which genes and environments influence each other, combining forces to shape our minds. In the latter parts of the lecture, we'll be focuses on specific genes, in fact, and their interaction with specific conflicts. After today's lecture, you'll have even further reason to pause before using the term "nature versus nurture," as it's truly nature and nurture, combining in intriguing ways, that shape our minds.

Last time we considered family studies, twin studies, and adoption studies; the core methods of behavior genetics. There's a standard model in this field called the "additive model" of behavioral genetics. This is an important model, because it's the basic one we've had for understanding how genes and environments work to shape individual differences in behavior for many years. Although it's the model most scientists go by, there are problems with it, which we'll come to appreciate as we discuss its key points and then try to transcend its premises. In this additive model, there are 3 main influences on variation in traits, behavior, and minds; and, quite importantly, they're all assumed to be independent of one another. The first influence, our focus last time, is genes. Again, from family, twin and adoption studies, we can estimate genetic contributions to individual differences in traits, behaviors, or disease states; the term is "heritability." But, as we discussed at the end of last time, heritability gets reified; there are a number of myths that we tried to dispel.

The second influence deals with the types of environmental influences that we usually think about when we consider context. These are what we called "shared environmental" influences. By this we mean those influences that any siblings in the same family experience similarly or share. For example, the effects of poverty tend to be shared by all family members, such as substandard housing, family stress, insufficient nutrition, etc. Or, of course, consider the parental discipline styles that families display: the authoritative, authoritarian, permissive, or neglectful parenting styles, which we discussed in some detail back in Lecture Nine. These environmental influences are what scientists believed to be the dominant influences on individual differences in minds for much of the last century.

Third, there is what we call "non-shared environmental influences," or sometimes "unique environmental influences." These refer to contexts that are different for different siblings; in other words, those that are experienced uniquely by each child in a family. This might be difficult to conceptualize initially, but think of it this way: Even in the same family, different children actually do have a lot of unique experiences. Each child has a different peer group, and different teachers. Even with respect to parenting style, parents may actually treat their different children quite differently; think, for example, of the parental "favorite," or the "black sheep" of the family. Furthermore, when children differ in age by more than a year or 2, there may be different economic conditions they experience or different neighborhoods, if the family moves; so, the neighborhood child one experiences at age 8 is really different from the neighborhood child 2 experiences at the same age.

This is called an "additive" model, because these 3 influences on individual differences are expected to add up to 100%. In other words, genes, shared environmental influences, and unique environmental influences are separate, and they must sum for the totality (100%) of explaining differences in behavior or traits. If genes explain everything—so that heritability is 100%—there's therefore no room left for shared or unique environment; conversely, if environment determines all the differences, there's nothing left for genes to explain, heritability would be zero.

What's happened with this model? When twin and adoption studies were used to obtain estimates for these 3 contributors to differences in the mind, especially during the explosion of research on this topic in the 1970s and 80s, some really unexpected results were revealed. First, as noted in our last lecture, the effects of genes on many traits and behavior patterns were, and still are, a lot higher than most people would have expected. Roughly half of the variability in most temperamental and certainly most personality traits in adulthood can be explained by genetic factors, as opposed to environments. The heritability of the "Big Five" personality traits—remember "OCEAN"; openness, conscientiousness, extroversion, agreeableness, neuroticism—ranges from about 40% to about 55%. The reasons why I thrive at parties and you are content with a rich inner life—maybe, actually, vice versa in truth—are at least half-related to differences in our genes.

A core implication is that it might be futile for parents to try to dramatically alter their children's temperaments or budding personalities. Remember instead the concept of "goodness of fit"; how the parent accepts, and more gently pushes and adapts, can be of great importance. The same is true for IQ scores across children: Somewhat over half of differences are related, overall, to genes; heritability of around 60%. Some have therefore argued that doesn't make much sense to make the attempt to raise IQ scores, which are as heritable as they are. But remember, the heritability of IQ is actually higher in the highest social classes, but far lower in the lowest classes. It's easy to reify heritability, unless we consider the many myths that exist about it; and IQ scores can be raised with intensive intervention.

For many traits well beyond IQ, including behaviors and emotional styles, genes matter relatively less and environments matter relatively more when environments are extremely unfavorable—malnutrition rampant in environment, lack of stimulation, abuse—or are extreme in such ways. Heritability tends to get lower when individuals experience contexts that are beyond the norm; because, again, heritability refers to the relative effects of genes versus environments, and if environments are extreme and variable, genetic effects (heritability) will decrease. Overall, though, the main finding is that genetic influences are stronger than we used to suspect.

What's the second core finding from behavior genetic research? Shared environmental effects are a lot smaller than we ever thought. For many traits—IQ, shyness, certain acting out and behavior problems—their contribution is 10%, maybe at most 20%. This is radical, if you think about it: All of the things we thought of as the primary influences on how the mind differs across members of our species—parenting styles, social class—explain relatively small amounts of the variation in most personality traits, in IQ scores, or other aspects of the mind and behavior. Even more, whatever shared environmental effects may be apparent for children tend to decrease by adulthood; so shared environmental effects don't persist over time, either. This may seem somewhat mystifying, but stay tuned a bit later for some explanation.

Third, also unexpectedly, non-shared or unique environments explain roughly similar amounts of variation as do genes, and in some cases, even larger. This is kind of radical, too; it appears to be the idiosyncratic, individualized experiences that determine much more of the differences across human minds than was believed or reported in many textbooks throughout much of the last century. Again, it's not how authoritative you are as a parent, it's the particular relationship you have with child A versus B. More than parenting, it may be the peer group to which each particular child belongs; certainly best friends, a big influence as we discussed earlier, differ between siblings.

As a result, traditional developmental psychology—some believe—should be spending less time on measuring "overall" parenting styles and more time on examining the particulars of a specific interactional pattern between parent and each particular child; so-called "permissive" parents being much stricter with one child than another. There's a technical point here: Non-shared or unique environmental influences might actually be somewhat inflated, because they include in their estimates errors in measuring environments and the thoughts and behaviors they influence. Difficulties in assessment might make the non-shared part of the equation somewhat larger than it otherwise would be. Even so, non-shared environmental effects are often unexpectedly big.

This overall pattern—larger effects of genes than we ever believed possible; much smaller effects of shared environment than we could have imagined; and often quite large effects of unique, idiosyncratic environments—rocked the scientific world, and indeed parts of popular culture, in the latter years of the 20th century; they really flew in the face of most conventional wisdom. Parents began to question whether their own parenting styles—these are supposedly the mainstays of shared environmental influences—really matter much at all. In fairness, recent evidence does reveal that shared environments do matter for certain kinds of problem behavior in children and adolescents. The clearest example is for aggression and antisocial behavior and delinquency; shared environmental may contribute up to 20% of individual differences here. Those negative and coercive family interactions that often characterize the development of aggression are real in their influence. Let's just look a bit deeper here. For some children with very severe aggressive behavior patterns, not only have insecure attachments often been present in early life, but parents show a blend of both authoritarian (very harsh and strict) and permissive styles (the parents really let the kid's behavior go until the

©2010 The Teaching Company.

child ups the ante, crosses the line, and then boom, harsh physical and emotional treatment).

Where do we go from here in explaining our minds and their development, and individual differences in minds? Is it all in the genes we're born with, and in unique, even random life experiences? Let's go back to the additive model: Let's recall again its contention that genes, shared environments, and unique or non-shared environments are each in their own orbits, independent of one another. But this belief has really been challenged; some of the findings are quite revolutionary. How could, in fact, genes and environments combine forces? The short answer is this: Certain genes and certain environments tend to go together, fueling each other across a person's development. Certain genes may exert their effects only—or largely—in certain environmental contexts. In this way, the additive model really breaks down, when we consider how genes and environments work together. Let's now be concrete about just how genes and environments can show such interplay, exploring the crucial concepts of gene-environment correlation and gene-environment interaction in some detail.

There are 2 main types of gene-environment interplay. The first is "gene-environment correlation." The best way to convey this concept is through some concrete examples; but here's an overview first: The genes passed along from parents to children are often quite linked with the environments in which the children find themselves or even create for themselves. It's really not as simple as the classic additive model would have us believe; namely, that genes and environments independently affect individual differences. Let's start with a puzzling fact: The heritability of many behavioral traits increases the older we get. This seems unbelievable at first; genes are genes, they don't change across an individual's life. What could be going on here?

The heritability of aggressive behavior is actually quite low in the infant and toddler years; remember: the most aggressive humans are those between one and 2 or 2 ½ years of age. But by adulthood, chronic aggression is at least 50% heritable, if not more. Again, how could this be? Think of it this way: Over time, our genotype, the behaviors it tends to produce, will tend to create certain expectations for our behavior and may land us with peer groups that encourage aggressive and antisocial actions, propelling us to certain kinds of behaviors that amplify the initial effects of those genes. Young children with strong tendencies toward aggression, assertion, and impulsivity may earn reputations for themselves, fostering fear and rejection from peers, further intensifying the very genetic tendencies initially leading toward aggression. There may also exist a kind of self-fulfilling prophecy for the child; he or she comes to view himself or herself as the kind of person for whom aggression really works.

With this specific example in mind, here are 3 specific ways in which gene-environment correlation can work: First, there's what we call "passive" gene-environment correlation. Here, genes that are common to both parents and children influence parenting behaviors or the homes parents build; so the environment in which the child resides potentiates the genetic effects. Let's be concrete: Think of a child with intelligent parents. As we discussed, IQ is moderately heritable, so some of the association between parent and child IQ is mediated by genes. At the same time, these types of parents are likely to have many books in the home, to speak more words with their children than other parents, and to promote good study habits in their offspring.

To digress for a moment, but I hope productively: Intriguing research has shown that children in such families—upper middle class homes—hear many more words during the day than do children of poorer, or less intelligent families. Findings have emphasized that children from such verbally-rich homes fare better developmentally, both in terms of long-term outcome and even at the level of the organization of their brains, with enhanced language processing areas.

Overall—back to gene-environment correlation—the environment created by the family is linked with parental IQ and therefore with the genes that are partly responsible for IQ. A genetic advantage in this case is associated with, correlated with, environmental opportunity; the child is passively the beneficiary of this "double enrichment" from genes and environment.

Next, there is what we call "active" gene-environment correlation. In this case, the child inherits tendencies from the parents that propel him or her to perform behaviors that accentuate the inherited traits. Let's use some fancier language: The child's heritable tendencies influence his or her selection of environments. An example might help here: Children born to parents with tendencies toward substance abuse and delinquency may be prone to sensation seeking and abuse substances themselves. Such experiences may further erode self-control and emotion regulation. In other words, the genes inherited from parents with these kinds of tendencies may drive the child to perform behaviors that get him or her into more hot water, leading to further risk for substance abuse, delinquency, and the like. Again, genes and contexts are linked; such a positive feedback loop is likely to increase and spiral over time.

The third process is what we call "evocative" gene-environment correlation: Here, the child's inherited tendencies tend to elicit responses from people around him or her—such as the family, school, or neighborhood—that accentuate existing vulnerabilities or strengths. Children born to withdrawn or shy parents often themselves have heritable tendencies to fear novel situations; recall the concept of reactive or inhibited temperament back from Lecture Eight. As we've emphasized several times, these tendencies in the child elicit or evoke protective responses from parents, which serve to accentuate the child's basic inhibition. The kind of clear, firm, yet supportive parental "pushing" that might have helped the child to overcome the inhibition simply doesn't take place. Instead, the child's heritable resistance and avoidance tend to elicit the kinds of responses from caregivers that reinforce the initial tendencies, because maybe the parents themselves have these same traits. "It's OK, honey, we don't have to go to that play date; let's just stay in the car and you can settle down." Those are the kind of responses that accentuate the initial tendency.

What's the important message about gene-environment correlation? Very specifically, separating genes and environments in the classic additive model isn't accurate. It's no wonder, actually, that heritabilities might increase over time: The effects of genes are enhanced because of environments that accentuate the genetic potential, and these positive feedback loops increase the longer the person lives, propelling the initial, genetically-mediated tendencies to new heights.

The second type of gene-environment interplay in many ways is even more striking. Here, we're talking about what is called "gene-environment interaction." By interaction here, we're discussing a statistical concept, not just 2 things interacting casually. Specifically, when 2 factors interact, statistically speaking, the effects of the first are quite different when the effects of the second factor are considered. This might sound confusing; it shouldn't be if you think of it this way. Let's take the example males versus females: Maybe for males, taking a certain medication produces reductions in a behavior pattern like anxiety; but for females, the medication actually increases the anxiety with increasing dosage. This is kind of radical interaction between sex—male versus female—and medication; the effects of medication depend on the sex of the research participant, they're actually the opposite in males versus females.

Back to genes and environments; think of it this way: Maybe different genotypes, or different alleles of a particular gene, show different effects in different environments. Let's be concrete here: As we've discussed throughout the course, in many cases 2 or more different alleles of a given gene can exist. These different genotypes may lead to differences in behavior. But what if it's the case that these differences show up only in certain environmental contexts? The work by psychologist Avshalom Caspi and his colleagues is very relevant here: His team has followed a New Zealand birth cohort of 1,000 individuals; these are all the individuals born in the city of Dunedin, New Zealand in the early 1970s. This group has been the subject of lots of important research on their developing minds.

One of their first articles of the Caspi group on gene-environment interaction examined the effects of different genes—different alleles—related to serotonin, and the outcome was the risk for developing major depression (which we'll return to in Lecture Eighteen). Two different alleles exist of a specific gene that codes for the serotonin transporter; this is the molecule that removes serotonin from the synapse. The gene, naturally enough, is called the "serotonin transporter gene." Recall from Lecture Two, this transporter molecule captures serotonin and brings it back into the presynaptic axon terminal; there's less of this neurotransmitter available in the synaptic cleft. One form of this gene predicts somewhat less efficient serotonin transmission (this is the allele we'll call "s") whereas the other form actually codes for more efficient serotonin transmission (that's the allele we'll call "S").

The first question is whether people with various combinations of these alleles—ss, Ss, or SS—have different rates of depression by their mid-20s. It might make sense that those with 2 copies of the "s" allele, with less efficient serotonin transmission, would have a higher risk for depression. The second factor is environmental and contextual: It's during childhood, whether individuals had experienced maltreatment; and during adolescence and early adulthood, the amount of stressful life events and deep loss events they experienced. Both of these were measured carefully. This was a longitudinal study, so information from parents, teachers, and the individuals themselves was collected about every 2 years or so throughout development.

It might be thought of in this case that maltreatment, adolescent and adult life events, or both would predict later depression. What do the results tell us? First, considered alone, the alleles of the serotonin transporter gene didn't matter very much at all. The different allele combinations—S/s combinations—didn't differentially predict risk for depression; there was a slight tendency for people with the "s" allele to have more depression. Next, considered alone, the life events—maltreatment or negative life events—did matter some; those adolescents and young adults with more negative events or early maltreatment had a somewhat higher risk of depression by their mid-20s. But here's the key finding: The genetic factor statistically interacted with the life events factor and the maltreatment factor such that the inefficient form of the serotonin transporter gene ("s") strongly predicted depression by age 26, but only in those individuals with high levels of negative life events or high rates of earlier maltreatment. Only those with at least one copy of the "s" allele were susceptible to negative life events. Unless the 2 factors, genes and environments, are considered together interactively, you could assume that the gene really didn't have much of an effect on depression, or that life events mattered only a little. But, in fact, genes mattered a lot when life was difficult. Let's state it the other way around: Life events make a crucial difference, but chiefly for those with certain genotypes.

There are other examples from this research group and other research groups, too: Certain alleles code for the MAOA gene; this is the enzyme in the presynaptic axon terminal that helps produce more or less high levels of certain neurotransmitters. Which gene (allele) you have for MAOA interacts with early maltreatment to predict delinquency; only one from of the genotype with early child maltreatment yields high rates of delinquency in adolescence. Only those, again, with less efficient dopamine and norepinephrine systems—coded by the allele—and maltreatment are end up with high risk for delinquency.

Another example: There are 2 main alleles of the COMT gene, which also relates to the efficiency of key neurotransmitters in the brain. It interacts with the experiential variable of marijuana use in early adolescence to predict risk for psychosis and schizophrenia-like behavior patterns; which we'll discuss, again, in a subsequent lecture. Again, neither factor alone had a big impact; but those with the riskier gene pattern were at risk for psychotic experiences only if they had begun marijuana use prior to mid-adolescence (they'd started smoking pot early).

In some very recent findings, maybe the most intriguing of all, we now know that some people with "risk" genes or vulnerable temperaments actually do better than those without them under certain environmental conditions. Here's an example: Infants with very difficult temperament between one and 2 years of age show particularly strong problem behavior when they're reared in poor-quality home environments, that's expectable; but infants with this temperamental pattern actually show particularly low rates of problem behavior when they're reared in very high-quality environments. Infants with easy temperament didn't show any differential effect of parenting and home life. In this case, a biological, genetically related factor like difficult temperament or high negative emotionality really might be what we call a "plasticity" factor; children with this style are most likely to do either really badly or really well, for better or for worse. The effect of temperament or of a genotype could switch completely from being a risk factor to even a protective factor as the context changes. The people most negatively influenced by stressors may be the same people who could gain the most from enrichment.

These kinds of findings are not always replicated, but they do enough to matter; and what a lesson here for the additive model: Genes matter, but only in certain environments or certain situations or contexts. The effects of genes and environments can be seen only when we examine how they act together.

What does all of this mean? The essential point from the lecture today is that the common dichotomy of nature versus nurture is outdated and, in fact, inaccurate. Nature and nurture combine in incredible ways to shape the human mind. Genes can be switched on or off by events outside the cell nucleus; indeed, by events in the environment, both biological and social. Genes and environments are in constant interplay; epigenetic factors, those beyond the configuration of DNA inside our cell nuclei, are critical for gene expression. The genes linked to depression—for example, the serotonin transporter gene we discussed—probably don't cause depression per se, but rather a vulnerability to depression.

Let's consider this last fact in a slightly different way: These genes may actually operate by making the individual more vulnerable to stress; in other words, the effect of this kind of gene is to make the person more responsive to the environment. There may not be a gene that "causes" depression per se, but rather some alleles make the person more reactive to life difficulties. We've really come full circle, haven't we? Separating genes and environments is inaccurate and problematic. We should be extremely careful of the phrase "nature versus nurture" once again, because nature is linked with, and interacts with, nurture in ways that go far beyond our standard models.

In the development of the human mind, biology and experience are inextricably linked, just in the way that they are in evolution by natural selection. The effects of an individual's genes—both a single gene and several genes in combination—are inseparable from environmental effects. This is big news, indeed, for everyone concerned with the human mind. Thanks for your attention to this complex and fascinating material.

Lecture Sixteen
The Abnormal Mind—What Goes Wrong?

Scope:

A strikingly high percentage of individuals develop 1 or more forms of mental disorder throughout their lifetimes. Far from being figments of the imagination or products of weak volition or will, mental illnesses are among the most impairing conditions on earth. Studying the ways in which the mind can "go wrong" tells us a great deal about the ways in which the mind can flourish, and vice versa. An initial question pertains to defining mental disorder. The search for objective, biological indicators of mentally disturbed functioning continues, but social and cultural factors are inherent in any definition.

Outline

I. A major question is whether mental disorders exist on a continuum with normal behavior or constitute separable, discontinuous categories. Evidence is accumulating that nearly all forms of mental disturbance exist on a spectrum—that is, they lie on a continuum with normal behavior.

   A. The prevalence of mental illness is high, yielding strong impairment.

   B. Across the world, the major forms of mental illness have remarkably similar prevalence rates, strongly suggesting biological and evolutionary rather than purely cultural roots.

   C. Severe mental illness, involving psychosis, serious substance abuse, or suicide attempts, affect 6% of the population. Moderate forms, which can also be debilitating affect an additional 20%.

   D. Levels of impairment are high: Risk for suicide, loss of economic productivity, devastation to close relationships, impaired parenting skills, deep shame, and high risk for being victimized are all involved.

E. The Global Burden of Disease studies reveal that several forms of mental illness—including schizophrenia, depression, bipolar disorder, obsessive-compulsive disorder, and substance abuse—are in the top 10 most disabling diseases on the planet, rivaling infectious diseases, cancer, heart disease, and HIV.

II. An essential issue is how we can define behavioral abmormality or mental illness. Several different models have been proposed over the years.

A. Statistical: Mental illnesses are behavior patterns that fall on the "tails" of the normal distribution or bell curve. Yet knowing where the cutoff lies for differentiating normal versus abnormal scores is usually arbitrary.

B. Social deviance: Behavior patterns that violate a given society's social norms are indicative of mental illness. Yet when we define mental illness on the basis of social deviance, there is a great risk of branding unpopular or politically controversial behavior as the product of an underlying disease process.

C. Moral: Here, it is not simply social deviance but moral violations that are branded as products of mental illness. Although this attribution is clearly made when religion dominates the ruling of a society, moral ascriptions still occur in modern, secular cultures.

D. Medical: Mental illnesses reflect disease processes operating at the level of the brain or mind.

E. Ecological/impairment: Mentally ill behavior does not result from either inner dysfunction or faulty environments but from a mismatch between person and context.

F. Harmful dysfunction: Proposed by Wakefield, it has an explicitly evolutionary perspective. For consideration as mental disorder, a behavior pattern must create harm and reflect an underlying dysfunction in a naturally-selected mental function.

G. Transactional: Borrowing heavily from developmental psychopathology, this model integrates the study of normal and atypical development. People with mental illnesses are not qualitatively different but lie farther out the bell curve of various dimensions of functioning and symptoms.

III. Trauma also has major implications for mental dysfunction.

    A. Trauma involves extreme environmental distress that can be life-threatening, literally or symbolically. In our conflict-laden world, trauma can involve war and torture, abuse, rape, environmental disasters, or exposure to violence.

    B. The human mind is configured to respond to trauma through several self-protective mechanisms, which may, unfortunately, compromise later functioning when the traumatic stressor is removed.

    C. Post-traumatic stress disorder (PTSD) is a major category of mental illness. It comprises 3 main areas of impairment, including hypervigilance and strong indicators of anxiety, numbness and avoidance, and re-experiencing of the event.

    D. Not all individuals exposed to life-threatening trauma develop PTSD, which is moderately heritable: genetic vulnerability exists for extreme reactions to trauma.

Suggested Reading:

A host of excellent textbooks on abnormal psychology exist: For example, Kring and Johnson, *Abnormal Psychology*. For a review of models of psychopathology, see Hinshaw, *The Mark of Shame: Stigma of Mental Illness and An Agenda for Change*, chap. 1.

Questions to Consider:

1. What are some reasons why mental illnesses have come to supplant many physical illnesses as the most impairing conditions a person might encounter during his or her lifetime?

2. Which of the definitions of mental illness offered in this lecture is most compelling to you, and why?

Lecture Sixteen—Transcript
The Abnormal Mind—What Goes Wrong?

Today we tackle a major conundrum: Why do some minds—too many, in fact—go off track or fail to thrive? This could sound like a straightforward question, but consider this: If we have been naturally selected for survival and reproduction, why would so many humans not be able to regulate their emotions at all well? Why are others unable to display rational thought, or do they have a proneness to hear sounds or see objects that are not present in the environment? Why are others so sometimes overwhelmed by anxiety and fear that they cannot meet the tasks of everyday life? Why can others not focus attention adequately or make adequate social connections with other people? Wouldn't, in fact, everything for which we have been naturally selected lead to adjustment and health, with only rare exceptions? But mental disorders are far from rare, so the conundrum is real.

For the next 6 lectures, we will explore more closely the relationship between normal, healthy functioning and abnormal, pathological functioning. This link can tell us a great deal about the origins of the human mind. First, let's deal with a core issue: Does mental disorder exist on a continuum with normal functioning, or are there truly separate categories, or separate entities, differing qualitatively from the rest of the population? This seemingly simple question is really anything but. The same can be asked for many physical conditions as well, but the answer depends a lot on one's perspective. For example: When is high blood pressure actually considered to be hypertension, a medical illness? Here, the underlying variable of blood pressure clearly forms a bell curve in the population, so it's kind of arbitrary where to draw the dividing line, as we will soon discuss with respect to the statistical model of mental disorder. But for some individuals with extremely high blood pressure readings, there truly are underlying genetic vulnerabilities, as well as complications with constitution of their blood vessels, that place them "off the continuum."

Here's an example related to the mind: We tend to define mental retardation on the basis of a person's IQ score, when the score is quite low; usually under 70, cutting off the lowest 2 or 3% of the population. In fact, most people with mild to moderate mental retardation—with scores in the 50s or 60s—appear to truly be on the far end of the same continuum as those with scores just above 70; in other words, they have parents with below-average intelligence, they are often impoverished, they may have malnutrition, and a host of other risk factors for mild to moderate mental retardation. But there's a much smaller group who typically have even lower scores—20s, 30s, 40s, 50s—who develop mental retardation largely because of specific genetic or chromosomal abnormalities; Down syndrome and Fragile X syndrome are the 2 most common, there are at least 200 other known genetic conditions. Although still on the IQ curve, these individuals actually do appear to have qualitatively distinct and different causal factors from the majority with mental retardation.

The question is this: Is physical or mental disorder continuous or dimensional, on the one hand; or is it discontinuous, categorical, on the other? The answer is really that it depends; it depends on how we conceptualize the problem or perhaps on how severe the underlying condition really is.

In physics, there has been huge debate over the centuries about whether light is a wave (smooth and continuous) or a particle (composed of photons, discrete bits or units of energy). Light actually has both wave-like properties and particle-like properties, depending on the scale of observation that's applied. In the sciences of the mind, mental disorder itself could be either continuous or categorical as well, depending on how and where we look. Indeed, the closer we do look, the more we realize that just about all of the mental disorders that we know of exist on a spectrum or continuum, with a number of intermediate steps or conditions in between someone with severe problems and the normal range. Even schizophrenia or autism, usually thought of as severe, qualitatively distinct diseases or entities, are now known to be spectrum conditions; they exist on a continuum. In schizophrenia, some individuals show paranoia and strange thinking, but not the full schizophrenia illness; in terms of autism, some children having language abnormalities or moderate social problems but not the full condition we call autism.

A key question this: Just how prevalent and how debilitating are mental disorders? Let's be specific: Severe mental illness, usually thought of as involving psychosis—hallucinations, delusions, and thought disorder (the subject of our next lecture), along with very serious substance abuse or suicidal attempts—affect about 6% of the population of the United States; that's 1 in 16. These figures actually appear to be pretty consistent around the world, too. Moderate forms of mental disorder—which, of course, can also be quite debilitating— affect another 20% or so. Here's an example: agoraphobia, the utter fear of being outside or in open places; or depression that falls short of suicidality but can still lead to major problems with physical health and social functioning. If we go up the continuum even further, there are milder forms of mental disorders, including fears and phobias that may not be quite as debilitating. If we add all these up, over 40% of the general public is affected by mental disorder at one time or another in their lifespan. Child forms of mental illness—which include learning disorders, ADHD, autism, anxiety disorders, and depression as well— are also highly prevalent, affecting about one-quarter of children and adolescents. There aren't small percentages, for sure. We'll have more to say about these high numbers a bit later in the course from an evolutionary perspective.

In addition, mental disorders bring on high levels of impairment, misery, and suffering. School failure, major problems with peer relationships, devastating loneliness; all of these often accompany mental illness in children and adolescents. In adults, we can count many forms of impairment: loss of economic productivity; devastation to close relationships; impaired parenting skills; often a sense of deep shame; a high risk for being victimized by others (that is, being a victim of violent crime). The stereotype is that mental disorders are inevitably linked to violent behavior in the individual; this is sometimes true, but on average, people with serious mental illness are far more likely to be victims of violent crime. Data clearly show that hundreds of billions of dollars are lost each year to the economy resulting from mental illness.

In terms of the most extreme impairment one can have, the ultimate self-destructive act, suicide: It is highly related to depression and bipolar disorder as we'll hear, but it can accompany schizophrenia or obsessive-compulsive disorder; this is the devastating pattern of obsessional thoughts of dirt or death, leading to compulsive rituals of cleaning or checking to ward off these obsessional fears. In sum, mental disorders are troublingly prevalent, and they often yield substantial impairment.

How do we know this? For many years, in fact, mental disturbances weren't taken as seriously as they should have been. After all, they were "mental" in nature, they're in the mind; many thought that they were malingering, or maybe products of weak personal effort or will. We can recall this from some of the less compassionate aspects of spiritual and humanistic models of the human mind.

During the 1990s, the World Health Organization (WHO) decided to take a numerical look at the impact of all illnesses across the world. To make a long story short, they composed a formula involving what are called "Disability Adjusted Life Years" (DALYs) to serve as an objective indicator of the actual impact of illness on productivity, time off work, time in the hospital, loss of wages, etc.; it's a complicated mathematical formula, as objective as possible. The first report using this formula was published in 1996, called the "Global Burden of Disease" study; it's been regularly updated by WHO since that time. The findings, back in 1996, were startling. Among the 10 most impairing illnesses on Earth, 4 were mental disorders: schizophrenia, depression, bipolar disorder, and obsessive-compulsive disorder. Today, depression has moved into the number 1 spot as the most impairing disease on Earth overall, given its prevalence and huge impact on physical problems—diabetes and heart disease, to name 2—and major life impairments. Alcohol abuse has joined this top 10 list as well. Mental illnesses, mental disorders, have come to equal or surpass infectious diseases, cancer, heart disease, and HIV as major sources of human misery and disability. With health economists asserting such on the basis of hard data, government leaders and the public have begun to listen more than ever.

We can't discount the huge impact of mental disorders; even in these hard economic terms, we can't discount them at all. But how to define what mental disorders are constituted of? How do they relate to the mind's strengths and powers? Can they be real or objective if they involve behavioral deviance, often defined in the context of certain cultures and cultural norms for behavior? Because they're called "mental," they must be just up in the mind. But a major advance, as we discussed in terms of brain imaging in Lecture Two: We can now visualize certain patterns of mental illness as part of the brain.

Brain imaging studies are starting to show us the realities of these conditions. At present, they aren't definitive enough yet to be used for a valid diagnosis; but public acceptance of the reality of mental illness has definitely increased with our ability to see now the multiple colors of an fMRI scan, of various brain regions that do and do not light up in correlation with certain illness categories. This is a fascinating case of the ability to counter dualism through brain imaging.

Several different ways of defining mental illness have been proposed over many years, even many centuries; discussing these models should reveal what we know, and what we don't know, about the origins of the troubled mind and linkages with healthy minds. The scientific question as the underlying nature of mental illness is perhaps one of the great questions that human beings have grappled with throughout the ages.

Let's start with a very common way of defining mental disorder: This is our first model, the Statistical Model. Here, mental illnesses may reflect behavior patterns that fall on the "tails," the ends, of the normal distribution or bell curve; so we're dealing with a continuum model here. Someone with too much, or too little, of a particular behavioral or emotional style would be considered literally "ab-normal"; that is, away from the norm, the mean, of the distribution. Two current examples: Depression and ADHD are typically defined from statistically rare scores on relevant rating scales. The most inattentive and overactive children—those in the top 5 to 7%, for example—may be considered for diagnosis on the basis of parent and teacher ratings. Self-reported symptoms of depression in adults are used often for that diagnosis.

Here are 2 core issues and problems: First, what's the cutoff point? Who's on one side of the boundary and who's on the other? For many forms of behavior—and, indeed, for many physical signs—the cutoff is certainly not written in stone. Let's go back to hypertension and high blood pressure as an example: It rose dramatically in prevalence in the summer of 2003 in the U.S. Why? Not because of a health problem, or suddenly more stress, or more salt in the diet; but because a change was made in the official standards for the levels of systolic blood pressure (that's the top number) and diastolic blood pressure (the bottom number) considered as either borderline or actual hypertension. Some traits behaviors that are not rare statistically: Let's take tooth decay. Where there's no fluoridation, 80% of children develop dental caries. Or to use a mental health example, child abuse: much more prevalent than we used to think; not statistically rare but quite problematic. If we define deviance solely on the basis of rarity, we might overlook some major problems that are staring us directly in the face.

Here's the second issue: In a true statistical model, there would be equal abnormality on both sides of the bell curve; it's as rare to be low on the continuum as high, in a statistical sense. But in actual practice, we consider only one side of the curve as "abnormal." We tend not to diagnose or treat people who have too little depression, or very little in the way of ADHD symptoms. In fact, the other side of the bell curve might be considered as a strength or asset; consider IQ scores: the high end is often considered gifted. The statistical model gives us a start, but we need more than statistical abnormality to define mental disorder validly.

Let's go to a second perspective: Here, in the social deviance model, mental disorder is thought to involve behavior patterns that are abnormal not statistically but with respect to social norms. Behaviors that violate a society's social standards may be considered indicative of mental illness. Back in the 19th century, the field of sociology in part began with this idea: Communities and societies cohere and stick together when and only when there are clear behavioral norms. Penalties for violating these norms reward the members of society who conform, forging a more cohesive social unit. There are big tendencies for all societies to notice and punish those whose behaviors violate social and sometimes legal norms. If we brand violators of such norms as mentally imbalanced or disturbed, something more comes into play, too: In this perspective, only people who are really "off" mentally—that is, only people who are irrational, disturbed, crazy, or mentally ill—could have even thought of violating the norms in the first place. The norms are really reified.

But when we define so-called "mental illness"—directly connoting a disease process inside the body and brain—on the basis exclusively of social norm violations, what's the risk? Of branding unpopular or politically radical or deviant behavior as the product of an underlying disease. This "illness" designation, again, discounts any social or political meaning of this behavior.

In the social deviance model, behavior patterns that are thought of as mentally ill in Society A might actually be quite adaptive and healthy in Society B. Recall in the former Soviet Union, there was a psychiatric diagnosis called "antisocialist personality"; anyone going against the tide of the government was certifiably mentally ill. The social deviance model is subject to extreme cultural relativity;

it doesn't satisfy those who would wish for some more objective, biological means of diagnosing and branding mental disorder, and it certainly can be used for politically repressive ends. But there may be something to the notion, in terms of natural selection of a species as social as ours, that some individuals who really can't work at all toward the social good could be problematic.

Third, there's the Moral Model; this is really an extension of the social deviance model into ethical and moral realms. In this case, mental illness is linked to violations of moral codes. Mentally ill behavior is explicitly considered to be morally weak or evil, or both. This attribution is most likely to be made when punitive religious beliefs dominate a society, but moral ascriptions may still occur in modern, secular societies, too. Let's give an example: Which day in modern history witnessed the most precipitous decline in the prevalence of mental illness ever? That was a day in the early 1970s, when the American Psychiatric Association by vote of its membership officially eliminated homosexuality from the official category of mental disorders. It had actually been in the *Diagnostic and Statistical Manual of Mental Disorders* prior to that time not because any longer of objective evidence for pathology, but because of lingering moralistic views.

Even today, with our emphasis on scientific, medical, naturalistic principles, it's good to question how much we intentionally—or even unintentionally—use a moral standard or perspective to consider substance abuse, or homelessness, or muttering or talking to oneself as flaws in behavior or moral fiber, linked to the loss of reason, another a key tenet of the humanistic model of the mind.

Let's move to number 4, the Medical Model; or as we should really say, in plural, the Medical Models. The idea here is naturalistic in perspective: Mental illnesses reflect disease processes operating at the level of the brain and then the mind. In current terminology, mental illnesses are often considered brain diseases—we see this in public service announcements—and, in fact, big new areas of new research are emerging right before our eyes. With these great advances in neuroimaging strategies, psychiatrists, psychologists, and the general public are now "seeing" the specific brain regions that may be involved in certain mental disorders. But again, with the complex interplay between biology and experience, and between genes and environments, it's not nearly so straightforward!

In fact, even in so-called physical medicine, there is not one single "medical model." There are, in fact, a variety of models related to infectious diseases versus chronic diseases versus what are now called multifactorial diseases—hypertension, cancer, and pulmonary diseases—which certainly have some genetic risk, but may be triggered by toxins, stress, or even lifestyle. These are now the leading causes of morbidity (illness) and mortality (actual death) in the world. In the typical medical model, we see the patient and look for "signs" (these are objective tests, maybe a fever measured with a thermometer) and "symptoms" (the patient's report of problems), and we'd like to see if they coalesce into "syndromes." A "syndrome" is a group of correlated symptoms, going together at the same time. But what we're really after are "disorders"; these are syndromes with a unifying cause. If I have fever, I'm achy, and lethargic, those are symptoms; and sometimes that combination could indicate a flu-like syndrome. But there could be an underlying disorder of viral meningitis, or bacterial meningitis, or pneumonia.

Perhaps the most significant issue in medicine as related to mental health is that in medicine, there are usually some objective markers of the underlying condition or disorder; a lab test to confirm that it really is bacterial and not viral. But this kind of objectivity doesn't exist yet for most forms of mental illness. Brain imaging studies are based on still-small groups of patients; not everyone with similar symptoms may end up showing the same neural "signature." Even somebody with a vulnerable genotype may develop a mental disorder only if he or she experiences certain environments; a key point raised in an earlier lecture.

Let's move now to model number 5, the Ecological or Impairment Model; here, it's the fit between the person and the environment that's crucial, just as it was in the "goodness of fit" concept in our discussion of temperament. What's the premise? Mentally ill behavior doesn't result from exclusively inner dysfunction or exclusively faulty environments, but from a mismatch between person and context. A very an active and inquisitive child in a very rigid classroom could result in a misdiagnosis of ADHD. A key implication here is that the "same" level of disturbance might be viewed as a mental disorder in Setting A, but could actually be viewed as adaptive in Setting B. The importance of this model is that it makes us quite aware of how important it is to examine the context in which behaviors take form. It makes it harder than ever to claim that all mental disorders are 100% biological or genetic in origin.

Here's model number 6: It was proposed by Jerome Wakefield, a mathematically and philosophically trained professor of social work, now at New York University. His view of mental disorder is based on evolutionary theory, so let's pay close attention. Harmful Dysfunction offers a dual criterion set for mental illness: Number one, mental disorders must yield harm and impairment. We wouldn't call anything a mental disorder illness unless the behavior patterns cause harm either to the self or others. Here's an interesting example: In medicine, there are some rare individuals who are born with 6, instead of 5, toes; this is the result of a rare genetic condition. But this really doesn't matter for the individual; there's no real harm, and it's not even listed in most indicators or indexes of physical disorders.

But harm alone isn't sufficient; we might be right back in the relativism of the social deviance model if harm were the only criterion. Wakefield says dysfunction is also required; the behavior pattern must yield harm, but also be dysfunctional. He means by this that from the perspective of natural selection and evolutionary psychology, some mental mechanism that has been shaped by evolution as a core mental function is not operating in a functional way. What about rational thought and our capacity for that; or the ability to perceive the world accurately? These are naturally selected mental modules, according to Wakefield; and if they aren't working properly, and if there's harm, then we could assert that a mental disorder is taking place. Hallucinations and delusions are examples of dysfunction in basic perception. Thought disorder signals a failure in rational thought; serious depression, a clear dysfunction in the ability to regulate negative emotion.

This model's intriguing: For the first time, evolution is explicitly part of the definition of mental illness. But the HD (or Harmful Dysfunction) model isn't yet perfect: We don't yet fully understand how natural selection has produced behavioral systems or mental modules, or how to define dysfunction in such systems. There's still the risk that one person's dysfunctional thinking could be another person's social deviance or political incorrectness. Still, the Harmful Dysfunction Model is a bold attempt to bring evolution into the picture.

Finally, number 7, there's what we call the Transactional Model. Borrowing from developmental psychopathology, and reflected in many of the earlier lectures from this course, the transactional model integrates the study of normal and atypical development. Here are some core assumptions: People with mental disorders are not qualitatively different, but simply lie further on the bell curve of various dimensions of functioning and symptoms. They often have periods of normal functioning, and share the same hopes, struggles, fears, and frustrations as anyone else. Mental disorders are not just social deviance or mental flaw, but they're not, also, solely medical or biological problems; they are deflections from normal developmental pathways. In fact, most forms of adult mental illness have their origins in childhood or adolescence, and most child and adolescent conditions extend into adulthood. It's likely to be in the complex interactions and transactions among genetic and contextual factors that we see how and where dysfunction occurs. Admittedly, this is a complex model, just as our course is complex; but it may be closer to the ultimate truth than some of the other, more simplistic models.

Our tour of these 7 definitional models reveals that each has something to contribute, but none is yet perfect or complete. Our science and our narrative abilities as a species still have a long way to go for us to get full understanding.

We're going to end today's lecture with one potential contributor to mental disorder: the experience of trauma. We define "trauma" as the exposure to extreme environmental distress that can be actually or symbolically life-threatening. In our conflict-laden world, trauma can involve war, torture, abuse, rape, environmental disasters, or exposure to violence, to name some of the most salient. The human mind appears to be configured to respond to severe trauma through several self-protective mechanisms, although they unfortunately may compromise later functioning even when the traumatic stressor is no longer present.

PTSD (post-traumatic stress disorder) is a major category of mental illness. Here are the 3 main symptom areas: First, hypervigilance, strong indicators of anxiety (startle); second, numbness and avoidance (this is keeping one's guard up; often isolation and being emotionally walled off); and third, re-experiencing of the event involuntarily through flashbacks or nightmares. These symptoms can be not only terrifying but also quite debilitating. Here's an important fact: Not all individuals exposed to such life-threatening trauma develop PTSD;

so the traumatic event is necessary, but it's really not sufficient for this condition to emerge. In fact, PTSD is has a moderate heritability: Genetic vulnerability exists for extreme reactions to trauma. We know this from studies of identical versus fraternal twins who have experienced trauma; identical twins are more likely to have concordance—in other words, to both develop PTSD—than are fraternal twins. But identical twins do not inevitably both develop PTSD, either; biology and experience interact.

Understanding the role of trauma in the mind's problems helps us to realize this: Genes and contexts do come together and interact in creating risk for mental disorder; this is a key theme to which we return in each of our next 4 lectures.

Overall, there's no clear consensus today on how to characterize mental disorder; but there's no doubting, either, its reality, its impact, and too often its tragedy. One of the great scientific endeavors of our current era, following centuries of debate and contention, is how to define what precisely constitutes mental illness.

In our next lectures, we will contrast the potential of the human mind with core dysfunctions and mental disturbances: rational thought versus schizophrenia, emotion regulation versus mood disorders, attention span and impulse control versus ADHD, and social connectedness versus autism. At that time, we'll be ready to understand how evolution helps us understand a key paradox: Mental disorders continue to exist, despite their levels of impairment and their moderate to high heritability. The material forthcoming is sometimes uplifting, sometimes tragic, but—at least in my view—always fascinating. Thanks for your continued attention.

Lecture Seventeen
Rationality, Psychosis, and Schizophrenia

Scope:

Although normal capacities for inferring reason and rationality are not always perfect, when the potential for rational thought and accurate perception is lost, devastation typically ensues. Schizophrenia is a disorder affecting 1% of the general population, with onset during mid- to late adolescence. This lecture covers the symptoms and impairments related to this highly impairing condition, its genetic and experiential origins, evidence about its neural underpinnings, the promise of both psychotropic medications and various forms of psychological interventions, and the ways in which understanding the schizophrenic mind can help us comprehend the development of rationality and personal identity in all of us.

Outline

I. The capacity for rational thought is believed to be a uniquely human ability.

   A. Humans' ability to perceive the outside world with accuracy enabled our survival amidst larger and faster competitors. Clearly, there was selection pressure on such traits.

   B. On the other hand, humans are imbued with a number of mental heuristics that do not always consider rational contingencies or long-term consequences.

II. Psychologists have distinguished 2 types of thinking: the first of which is highly intuitive, reflexive, and automatic, yet prone to errors; the second is controlled, effortful, and judicious, yet costly in terms of mental energy.

   A. When one has lost the capacity for the second type of reasoning and thinking, unable to perform careful analysis of long-range consequences, functioning is likely to be severely compromised.

   B. At times, a lack of clear perception or rational thought, including primary process thinking propels artistic and spiritual experience.

C. Overall, when distorted perceptions and irrational thought processes cannot be controlled, devastation may result.

III. Psychosis is a syndrome, a constellation of associated behaviors, involving major problems in perception, rational thought, and behavior control.

A. A core feature is hallucinations, which involves perceptions of sights, sounds, aromas, and sensations of touch in the absence of external stimuli. Auditory hallucinations are the most common.

B. Delusions are prominent; these are fixed, false beliefs that are impervious to counterargument. These can be grandiose, self-deprecating, or sometimes quite bizarre Paranoid delusions increase the potential for the individual's aggression.

C. Formal thought disorder, a breakdown of the logic of thought, is marked by associations that are loose, meandering speech, and a breakdown of reason.

D. Agitation and loss of contact with reality are also part of psychosis in many cases.

E. A syndrome may have multiple origins. Psychosis is associated with severe mania or depression, advanced stages of HIV infection, extremely high fever, sensory deprivation, and to the disorder termed schizophrenia.

IV. Schizophrenia is a condition documented throughout history and in every culture, which involves periods of psychosis, along with or alternating with deficit symptoms—low motivation, loss of pleasure, social isolation, restricted or unusual affect.

A. Approximately 1% of the world's population has schizophrenia, with nearly equal rates in each nation.

B. In some cases, symptoms wax and wane; in other cases, the clinical presentation is chronic.

C. The impact of schizophrenia on individuals and families is devastating, with nearly all areas of life functioning negatively affected.

D. Although families were blamed, for much of the 20th century, for causing schizophrenia via negative or intrusive parenting, the heritability of schizophrenia is substantial (50–60%). Recent evidence reveals that deletions of genetic material from chromosomes may be involved in some cases. Prenatal and perinatal complications may also play a role.

E. A number of brain systems and regions are implicated in schizophrenia: Dopamine-containing neurons projecting from the midbrain to the frontal cortex are implicated in psychotic symptoms; the so-called deficit symptoms appear to involve multiple brain regions, including frontal lobe regions.

V. There are a range of developmental manifestations and impairments related to schizophrenia.

A. Schizophrenias typical age of onset is in the mid- to late teen years or very early adulthood. It is unknown if hormonal surges of adolescence, the identity issues confronting adolescents, drug use, or some combination of these and other factors trigger the onset.

B. Studies reveal that schizophrenia can be predicted from observations made during infancy and toddlerhood. Children who later develop schizophrenia, contrasted with a control group, reveal abnormalities of motor behavior and unusual emotional responses many years before the classic symptoms of schizophrenia emerge.

C. Although many symptoms do persist, only a minority of those with schizophrenia have chronic forms. Improvements can and do occur in many cases.

VI. Treatments for schizophrenia involve medications that influence dopamine and other neurotransmitters, as well as rehabilitation-oriented psychosocial treatments focused on social skills, vocational training, and family support and education.

A. The first generation of antipsychotic medications, originating in the 1950s, blocked a certain postsynaptic receptor for dopamine. A new generation of these medications, which can target deficit symptoms as well as psychosis, acts in different ways, on both dopamine and serotonin.

B. One-on-one psychotherapy designed to foster insight has not proven very successful for schizophrenia, but family-based treatments designed to reduce negative interactions and conflict, as well as behavioral interventions intended to promote social and vocational skills, have proven effective.

C. At present, the key objective is on rehabilitation rather than cure.

VII. When the capacity for rational thought is severely compromised, the condition called schizophrenia is a devastating consequence.

Suggested Reading:

Many psychiatric journals contain the latest research on schizophrenia, including *Schizophrenia Bulletin*. One of the best and most accessible books on the topic is Gottesman, *Schizophrenia Genesis.*

Questions to Consider:

1. How can one tell the difference between rational thinking, thinking that is unpopular or radical, and thinking that is truly irrational and disordered? What standards are helpful in making such distinctions?

2. Schizophrenia involves both psychotic features and negative/deficit symptoms. What are the ways in which each type of symptom is disabling for individuals with this condition?

Lecture Seventeen—Transcript
Rationality, Psychosis, and Schizophrenia

The key theme for our next 4 lectures is the relationship between the mind's abilities and powers on the one hand, and its disorders and pathologies on the other. Today we feature the mind's capacity for accurately perceiving the world, for rational thought, and for high-level executive control, which are some of the mental functions most crucial for performing everyday tasks that ensure our survival. After all, how would we fare in our lives without accurately representing the world; without thinking strategies that are abstract, clear, and grounded in reality; and without that core ability to inhibit previously rewarded responses when we sense that a better strategy might actually be more advantageous?

None of us always perceives the world with complete accuracy, nor do we always reason perfectly well; in fact, understanding some of these normative ways in which we don't behave or reason with accuracy can give us some clues as to the evolutionary origins of our minds. But when accurate perceptions and rational abilities break down utterly, life can really be a struggle. Indeed, one of the most devastating mental illnesses in existence, called schizophrenia, is intimately involved with breakdowns in perception, rational thinking, and higher-order executive functions.

To start, we've discussed extensively in earlier lectures that our species was under selection pressure to be able to perceive our surroundings with a high degree of accuracy. But acts of visual perception aren't simple one-to-one correspondences of the "real world" into our brains. Our eyes take in information from slightly different angles and the visual centers devote billions of neurons every waking moment to the task of representing the world in a 3-dimensional way. But we don't simply "copy" the world; acts of perception are active constructions.

For auditory perceptions, the middle and inner ear transduce sound waves into signals that end up in our auditory cortex in the temporal lobe to represent the incredible aural phenomena all around us; this is an equally spectacular feat. Think of the rich tones and overtones we constantly hear, how we can track location and distance, and how everything from the calls of predators or mates, along with symphonies of sound, enrich our experience. Hearing promotes both survival and provides experiences regarding the deepest parts of our humanity. Other hallmarks of our mind are the capacities for rational thinking, at least some degree of accurate self-reflection, and the performance of high-level executive functions.

But let's pause: A fascinating line of research, which is a subfield of cognitive psychology sometimes called "judgment and decision making," examines the ways in which humans often make regular errors about the world. If most of us are offered a choice to get $50 today versus $100 in 6 months—the latter is a really good interest rate—most of us would choose the former. This is called, formally, a kind of "temporal discounting"; we take the immediate, rather than calculate the longer-term gains over time. We also tend to be swayed by catastrophe, risk, and the potential for negative outcomes; it's as though the potential for something to go really wrong outweighs stronger evidence that something really might go right. In addition, we're often pulled in by the personal and the immediate, rather than more calculated, long-range consequences of our actions. This is why, some cognitive psychologists would argue, we are so concerned with the plane crash—very rare statistically, but salient and visceral to us today—but not the long-range consequences of, for example, failing to be more energy efficient or maintain the planet's health, which may save many more lives in the long range.

We also tend to predict the future based on information that's readily available to us, rather than using harder-to-find but important information that may could be more stable or representative. We tend to take the easy way out—"Well, I know a guy who got sick because he lived near power lines"—rather than the more accurate, more complex kinds of calculations that might prove more valid. This is called the "availability heuristic"; we tend to use information that's readily available to us.

These are examples—what I've just been talking about—of what are sometimes called mental "heuristics"; these are rules of thumb we all tend to use for thinking about the world. More deliberate thought might lead to other in some ways more accurate "construals," but we tend to use these heuristics. The bottom line is this: Sometimes these heuristics and rules of thumb are quite biased, leading us to inaccurate conclusions. Why would we do this when a more careful, cautious, "reasoned" analysis might help us to see the situation more rationally?

Think of evolution and the contexts in which early humans developed: Social groups were relatively small (150 at most), danger lurked everywhere, and quick decision making, often on the fly, was called for. Those humans—let's take an example—who made a decision that a stick, seen quickly in peripheral vision, was really a snake would have been alarmed and frightened unnecessarily, but they're not really the worse for wear. But what about those who mistakenly thought the opposite, that the snake was just a stick? They may not have survived long enough for their genes to propagate. Tendencies to personalize inanimate objects and to anticipate dire consequences in ambiguous circumstances were clearly the subjects of positive selection pressure.

What I'm talking about here reflects what is sometimes called Strategy 1 versus Strategy 2, or Type 1 versus Type 2 thought strategies. A lot of people have contributed to this view; Princeton psychologist and Economics Nobel Laureate Daniel Kahneman, who received his doctorate at Berkeley and who taught with us in our department for many years, is a core proponent. In short, Strategy 1 thinking is automatic, quick, reflexive, and quite intuitive; but, again, prone to these kinds of heuristic errors. This kind of thinking was clearly shaped by natural selection, and is usually our default because of the sheer numbers of stimuli we encounter, the decisions we have to make every day, and the huge energy levels required to kind of go beyond it. On the other hand, Strategy 2 thinking is highly effortful, laborious, and very calculated. We often reserve this for situations where a lot of deliberation and considered thought is needed to escape some of the biases of our usual, Strategy 1, intuitive mode. We tend to use Strategy 1 thinking most of the time; it's easier and quicker and often guides us well. But we need to use Strategy 2 strategies to think through all the angles of a situation; this is clearly a uniquely human skill, as far as we know.

Despite these mental shortcuts and heuristics—which do tell us something about the evolutionary conditions under which we emerged as a species—the ability to use effortful processing, to think rationally when truly needed, and to use all of our executive functions really keep us on our path to survival. Such functions, mediated by the frontal lobes and their intensive interconnections with other parts of the brain, are a crowning achievement of our human capacities. But here's a provocative question: Are these abilities always what we really want? Sometimes ultra-clear perception or ultra-rational thought may be too stiff or too stilted. What we sometimes term "primary process" thinking—this is a term that Freud used—in which images blur and associations are not always logical or linear may actually help to propel artistic, poetic, and spiritual experience. The key is that the person is able to harness these aberrant perceptions and cognitions and resynthesize or reintegrate them.

In truly creative thought, it's sometimes important to be able to let go of our usual tight control, as long as we can recover it. Here's an example from the world of art; and I think of some of Van Gogh's late self-portraits, in the latter years of his short life. His mental faculties were clearly deteriorating—many experts consider that he did, in fact, suffer from some sort of psychotic disorder—and we begin to see, in some of his self-portraits, a very wavy, intense background and very rushed, coarse brushstrokes. But even in these somewhat less realistic, less "rational" works, we can see that he maintained incredible control. In fact, these paintings are all the more poignant, revealing the huge conflicts in his mind with his clarity of vision still shining through. Back when I was in my 20s, making a tour of Europe on my own, I read a catalogue about Van Gogh's paintings, looking at them in several museums, and I remember the wording: "Art can go no higher," the catalog said, related to this ability to maintain control in the face of clear mental unrest.

On the other hand, when distorted perceptions and irrational thought processes cannot be brought back under control, devastation can result. This brings us to our concept called "psychosis." Psychosis is a syndrome; remember from the medical model. It's a constellation of correlated behaviors that tend to come together in the same person at the same time. Here, there are big issues in perception, rational thought, behavioral control, and insight. Here are the core symptoms of a psychotic episode: First, there are distortions in perceptions, which can culminate in hallucinations when we actually perceive stimuli that aren't out there in the real world. These typically start as exaggerations of real perceptual objects—the wind coming through the windows at night, the rustlings of paper—these can become distorted and magnified, and a bit terrifying. Actual auditory hallucinations, though, involve hearing sounds and voices in the absence of any sound waves coming from a real voice. This is not just hearing one's own thoughts aloud—a lot of us have that experience—but the sense that actual voices are talking to you or about you.

Hallucinations can occur in any modality, not just hearing. Auditory hallucinations are the most common, but visual hallucinations occur: seeing visions often associated with drug use, drug withdrawal, or certain kinds of brain injury; and so there are sights that we see in our occipital lobe and in our mind, but in the absence of any stimulus in the actual visual field. More rarely, tactile hallucinations can exist: the perception of touch or some skin irritation. A really terrifying one of these is the sense of bugs crawling under one's skin following ingestion of certain drugs or during alcohol withdrawal. People may—it's sort of horrifying to think of—pick at their skin until serious lesions occur in order to get rid of the supposed bugs or pathogens. Taste, or gustatory, hallucinations can also occur; and even olfactory hallucinations: smelling things that aren't actual odorants in the air. This could seem pretty obscure; but, in fact, olfactory hallucinations—for example, of one's own decaying flesh—can be terrifying perceptual experiences that can accompany schizophrenia or, what we'll talk about in our next lecture, mixed-state bipolar disorder.

These extraordinarily heightened perceptions, intriguingly, activate the same parts of the brain as real perceptions—we now know this from fMRI studies—so there's a misinterpretation of some internally-generated stimuli as emanating from out there in the world. A lot of researchers are investigating how such misattributions come into being.

Here's the second feature of psychosis, which we call "delusions." These are fixed, false beliefs that are very unusual sometimes and are almost always completely resistant to being argued out of. Many people have unusual or unpopular ideas, we don't want to label those as psychopathological; but in delusions, the person is the utterly convinced of this very unusual thought or belief, but often without a lot of emotion. Most people who thought, for example, that they were receiving radio transmissions from another planet in their head would be quite emotional indeed.

Some delusions are grandiose: When manic, a person may believe that he or she was placed on the world for a special purpose. Some delusions are self-deprecating: In serious depression, a person may believe that he or she is really guilty for the state of the economy or other world troubles. Some delusions are actually bizarre: again, the belief that a radio transmission is going through one's head from another planet. Some delusions are paranoid: the belief that other people are out to attack oneself. Of course, these would increase the potential for the individual to be aggressive as a kind of preemptive striking out against those threatening forces.

Here's a third feature of psychosis called "formal thought disorder." This isn't formal in the sense of tails and gowns; it means a breakdown in the form or structure of thinking, whereas delusions signaled a breakdown in the content of thinking, which we just discussed. In formal thought disorder, thinking is illogical; associations between ideas are jumbled and blurred; speech tends to meander through many twists and turns; sometimes unique words are formed, new words; and reasoning breaks down.

Here's an example, which I've composited from several individuals with clear signs of formal thought disorder:

Because, in peculiarity, I believe you suffer from the Oedipal Complex, to which I am an expert, as I remember your having made fun of my elderly state while I made normal pedestrianism on the sidewalk. . . Therefore, the complete duality of polarity related, of that sound going from one extreme to the next would be too much to hope for in a real evaluation, although these dynamics are not reflected on a minute by minute contemporaneous socio-political state, the former a microscopic true perspective of little relevance to the crowd tending against individuals, the latter an inverted, or upside-down microscope looked through backwards.

Try as you might, it's really just not possible to see coherent links across these ideas.

The fourth feature of psychosis often is "agitation"; the person is "wound up" very tightly, it might be expectable for someone with some of these other symptoms. Behavior, not surprisingly, becomes quite dysregulated.

Finally, when people are psychotic, they typically have very little insight; they're not aware that things are seriously amiss. In fact, people believe that others, or other powers, are affecting them. What's the core point here? There's very little motivation for change, because the locus of the problem is out in the world, not inside.

From our lecture on the medical model: Syndromes may have multiple origins or causes. In fact, in terms of the syndrome of psychosis, what are the triggers? Somebody with very severe mania or severe depression can become psychotic. People in advanced stages of HIV infection have psychotic symptoms. If the fever gets high enough—not exactly clear; 105, 106, 107, very dangerously high—psychotic symptoms can emerge. People who overdose on amphetamines or cocaine show many psychotic features; similarly, withdrawal from alcohol or sedative medications or drugs can lead to psychosis. If we had a long period of utter sensory deprivation, or if we went without sleep for a long period of time, most of us would begin to show some psychotic experiences. As frightening and disorganizing as these symptoms I just noted can be, all of us could well experience them under certain conditions.

But psychosis is also a core feature of the disorder we call "schizophrenia." Let's define this condition: This is a disorder documented throughout history and in every culture known; it's really universal. It's relatively rare, compared to depression (which we'll talk about next time); the lifetime risk of developing schizophrenia is about 1% of the population worldwide. What does it involve? First, there are often periods of psychosis, which we just defined; these are called the "excess" symptoms of schizophrenia. Then, periods of what are called "deficit" or sometimes "negative" symptoms can also occur; they may alternate with the psychosis or sometimes accompany it. These features include extremely low motivation, a severe loss of pleasure, social isolation, and either very restricted or quite unusual mood and affect.

Typically, after a period of psychotic behavior, which may—even without treatment—start to lessen or remit, many people with schizophrenia experience a period, even a prolonged one, of low energy; something we call "alogia" (very impoverished speech); a desire to be alone and keep away from others; and blunted, flat, or strange affect. These negative or deficit symptoms are quite disturbing to interaction partners; the individual appears preoccupied with inner thoughts, may describe highly unusual experiences without any apparent emotion, for example, laughing when describing attending a funeral. For a long time, we thought that these deficits indicated clearly that people with schizophrenia didn't really experience deep emotions in the way that most humans can and do. But my Berkley colleague, psychologist Ann Kring, has done very important work showing this: People with schizophrenia don't show on their face very much emotion—as much as others do—but their own subjective reports, and even their underlying physiology in their bodies, reveal that they are, in fact, experiencing the emotion inside.

What does "schizophrenia" literally mean? From the Greek, it means "split mind." This really means "a splitting of thought and affect" from the people who originated the concept, but it's not the same as a split or multiple personality, which we now call "dissociative identity disorder." Unfortunately, far too many people, otherwise knowledgeable, make this mistake, sometimes inadvertently—"That play had a schizophrenic plot, with contradictory images and messages"; "The weather was really schizophrenic today"—or sometimes in really demeaning fashion. Not too long ago, a manufacturer put out an advertisement about the "world's first schizophrenic lawnmower," which had 3 different functions for cutting, edging, and mulching; this is inaccurate, and also quite degrading. Again, the actual meaning of the "split" in the term "schizophrenia"—as defined by the Swiss clinician Eugen Bleuler a century ago—is a cutting off or separation of certain mental functions from one another and from the emotions.

What do we know about this devastating disorder called "schizophrenia?" The typical age of onset is late adolescence; this is right at the time of life when identity should be consolidating and relationships deepening. The original name given to this constellation of problems at the beginning of the 20th century was another Greek term, *dementia praecox*, which translates as "loss of cognitive abilities with early or precocious onset." Rarely, schizophrenia can begin at age 6, 7, or 8 in childhood; when it does, the long-term outcome is not at all favorable. Across the world, men and women are about 50/50 likely to develop schizophrenia, as are individuals from all ethnic and racial groups.

Schizophrenia tends to cluster the lower down the socioeconomic spectrum one goes. This could be because poverty is a risk factor for the development of schizophrenia, or it could be because people who develop schizophrenia tend to drift downward into lower social strata because of losing jobs and employment abilities as a function of these devastating symptoms; or both forces could be at work. In some cases, symptoms wax and wane over time. People have paranoid, psychotic periods; but even when these have cleared up, there's often a residual degree of negative or deficit symptomatology. In other cases, the clinical presentation is more chronic and long lasting.

Overall, the impact of schizophrenia on individuals and families is often devastating; all areas of life functioning are negatively affected. Again, right at the cusp of adulthood, individuals fail to be interested in work or relationships, become preoccupied with paranoid psychotic fantasies, and fail to show anywhere near their usual energy, drive, and pleasure in life. Unemployment, failure to finish school, a kind of long drifting period, and—in severe cases—chronic homelessness can result.

It's hard to imagine that there could be much "good"—in the sense of natural selection—that could emanate from this devastating cluster of symptoms. But in Lecture Twenty-One, we'll look back to evolutionary theory to help resolve this paradox: how a disorder like schizophrenia could be as devastating as it is, and as heritable as it is, yet still persist in our population.

What causes schizophrenia? Families were the direct culprits for much of the 20th century, blamed as having caused this disorder. In fact, there was this theory of the "schizophregenic" mother: intrusive, negative, hostile, prompting a retreat from reality in her son or daughter. But we now know that genetic influences are strong, rather than childrearing per se. There is a true schizophrenia "spectrum"; some individuals have the full symptom picture, but others related in the same families might have some degree of symptoms. Overall, the heritability of schizophrenia—this is this important concept from past lectures, how much individual differences are contributed to by genes—is nearly 60%; so there's a huge genetic liability. The more closely related one is to someone with schizophrenia biologically, the higher the risk of having the condition; identical twins have a much higher concordance than fraternal twins. But, as we discussed in our myths about heritability, there's not a single gene for schizophrenia, probably not even just a few; it's truly a polygenic condition, with multiple genes likely to be interacting with them and with the environment. In some rare cases, we know that schizophrenia is related to major copying errors, a deletion of whole chunks of DNA during meiosis.

Environments can accentuate the risk. A very intriguing study was done by Irv Gottesman, the noted geneticist from Minnesota and then University of Virginia. He studied identical twins (monozygotic twins) who are discordant for schizophrenia; one had it, and the other didn't (very interesting research design). In just about every single instance, the infant who was born second, was born at a lower birth weight, or who had more birth distress was the one who developed the disorder, as though the genes interacted and correlated with the environment in creating schizophrenia. Interesting research from Finland reveals that it's a combination, actually, of biological and genetic risk, plus some very discordant communication in the family home that is the big trigger of many forms of psychotic behavior.

Lots of brain regions and brain systems are implicated in this condition: Dopamine-containing neurons linking the striatum to the frontal cortex are linked to psychotic symptoms. The so-called "negative" or "deficit" symptoms involve multiple brain regions, including the frontal lobes. Elaine Walker, psychologist at Emory University, did some really interesting research with home movies. These were tapes and Super-8's made a number of years ago by families of their children's first birthday parties and other early life events. Some of the children later developed schizophrenia, and she recruited a control group of people with the same tapes whose children did not later develop schizophrenia. Observers carefully and "blindly" coded these tapes. Those infants and toddlers with somewhat abnormal motor behavior (gross motor movements) and unusual emotional responses were the most likely to show schizophrenia 15–20 years later. What's intriguing developmentally is how these problems in infancy and toddlerhood reemerge with a vengeance in new forms much later in life, following a gap in which the symptoms weren't too noticeable; there are some intriguing developmental processes undoubtedly going on.

Does schizophrenia inevitably accompany a person throughout life? Many symptoms do tend to persist, often waxing and waning; but only a minority of people with schizophrenia have truly chronic, lifelong forms. Improvements can and do occur in many cases; rehabilitation is possible, if not yet a cure. With strong encouragement and a structured approach to life, often with medication treatment, many individuals with schizophrenia can do quite well, defying the stereotypes. We could ask Elyn Sachs, a professor at the University of Southern California, whose book, *The Center Cannot Hold: My Journey Through Madness*, goes far in telling the truth about the pain of this condition that plagued her from early adolescence; but it also defies stereotypes, given her clear success in life. In other cases, however, of extremely chronic schizophrenia where the person has a large number of these deficit symptoms, what does brain imaging reveal? Actually, that the ventricles of the brain—those open spaces filled with cerebrospinal fluid—are enlarged, signifying that in those cases an actual atrophy of key brain tissue has developed.

How do we treat this condition? Many forms of treatment have been tried over the years. The most evidence today accrues to 2 forms of intervention: medications that influence dopamine and other key neurotransmitters in the brain; and rehabilitation-oriented psychosocial treatments focused on social skills, vocational training, and family support and education to reduce conflict and stress. In fact, there isn't much evidence that classic one-on-one therapy, dealing with emotional conflicts, does much to improve schizophrenia; and, in fact, highly unstructured dynamic therapies might actually be harmful, promoting a lack of structure and psychotic thinking.

The so-called "first generation" of antipsychotic medications, which began in the 1950s, blocks the postsynaptic receptor for dopamine. There's a newer generation of these medicines, sometimes called the "atypical" or "second generation" antipsychotic meds, which work both on dopamine and serotonin, and perhaps glutamate as well. We don't know precisely how they exert their effects. There's some evidence that they're more helpful than the first-generation class of meds for the negative/deficit symptoms. On the other hand, marked weight gain and even diabetic symptoms can result in some cases. No potentially effective treatment for any condition, medication or psychological, is without some potential for harm. Family-based treatments, which are designed to reduce negative interactions and conflict, and behavioral interventions designed to reward social and vocational skills, are also effective.

We don't yet know precisely why schizophrenia tends to develop in this key period of late adolescence. Is it a set of genes that suddenly get switched on at this key period of development? Is it a cumulative, transactional process involving genetic risk and some sort of ongoing life stress? But the lesson here is this: The consequences of not being able to display rational thought, or clear perceptions, or executive functions can be absolutely devastating. The more we know about executive functions, emotion, adolescence, the brain, and healthy environments—crucially, how these all develop—the better chance we have of preventing the negative consequences of this key disorder.

There are limits to constant ultra-rationality, and we humans have evolved a set of mental heuristics that are not always deliberative or accurate. Indeed, it may well take narrative understanding through exploring many different people's life experiences, and not just the results of objective science, to convey this essential picture of the humanity in all of us. But when a person loses the capacity for accurate perception of the world, rational thinking, or executive functions, serious impairment is likely to ensue. What's a core goal for future scientists, clinicians, humanitarians, and indeed all of us? It's to understand just how debilitating this symptom picture can be, but to realize that there is a fundamental humanity inside all such individuals.

The more we learn, the more we realize that even though chronic schizophrenia would appear to be a truly categorical entity off the charts—off the continuum of normal behavior—many components of this condition exist right on the same dimensions of rationality versus irrationality, and accurate versus inaccurate perceptions of the world, which we all share. Human rationality, far from being all-or-nothing, seems to be a wide spectrum, even within each individual.

Lecture Eighteen
Emotion Regulation and Mood Disorders

Scope:

Mood states give flavor and meaning to the events of our lives. Yet when emotion regulation fails and mood is persistently low, major depression may be apparent. Depression is now the most impairing illness on Earth, related to its high prevalence and its serious risks for impairment, loss of economic viability, and suicidal actions. When depressions are linked with manic episodes a condition called bipolar disorder, or manic-depressive illness, emerges. This lecture discusses the differences between normal fluctuations of mood and those implicated in mood disorders, reviews relevant gene-environment interplay, examines outcomes of medication and psychotherapeutic treatments, and probes the fascinating linkages between creativity, productivity, and mania.

Outline

I. We must first differentiate emotions that spanning several seconds; moods, which may last hours, or longer; affective styles; and mood disorders.

   A. All humans respond similarly to inherently pleasurable or inherently aversive stimuli with emotion displays of happiness or interest versus sadness, disgust, anger, or fear. Emotion displays span a few seconds in length. There is more universality than cultural relativity regarding emotion.

   B. Moods span hours or days. A positive or negative mood state triggers related cognitions and memories.

   C. Affective styles are predominant tendencies toward optimistic verses pessimistic appraisals of the world; they undoubtedly emerge from temperamental precursors during the earliest years of life.

   D. Mood disorders are syndromes involving multiple symptoms; they yield substantial impairment.

II. Depression is a term with multiple meanings—it can signify sad or pessimistic mood, as well as a syndrome involving not only a sad mood but altered sleep and appetite, negative thinking patterns, low motivation, self-reproach, and loss of pleasure.

A. A key trigger for a constellation of depressive symptoms is the experience of a loss—departure or death of a loved one, or symbolic losses such as experiencing a failure.

B. Depressions are likely to recur, in a condition called unipolar depression. Once one has had a major depression, there is a greater than 50% chance that more episodes will occur. After 2, odds of subsequent depressions are even higher.

C. Depression is surprisingly prevalent, especially in adolescent girls and women; it is a major source of significant life impairment.

D. Depression's costs relate to social support, contacts are initially supportive but then often get resentful; education and jobs; relationships; and suicide risk.

E. More women than men attempt suicide, but more men complete suicide, because of their use of more lethal means. Suicide risk is highest when a person is beginning to recover from a depressive episode: The energy is now present to perform the act.

F. In terms of causation, major depression has a moderate heritability—30% for men, 40% for women. Crucially, gene-environment interactions appear to play a key role—e.g., inefficient serotonin genes interacting with child maltreatment or adolescent/young adult negative life events.

III. Several models for explaining depression have been offered.

A. In psychoanalytic models, depression is the turning inward of the anger one feels in response to the departed person or ideal.

B. In social learning and cognitive models, the emphasis is on low levels of behavioral activation and the negative, ruminative thinking patterns that frequently accompany depressions.

C. Biological models incorporate inefficient or unregulated neurotransmission involving serotonin, norepinephrine, or both.

D. For unipolar depression, medications and specific forms of psychotherapy are both effective in cutting episodes short, and the combination of medication and therapy is optimal.

IV. Mania is a mood state beginning with expansive, elated mood, which often expands to later stages that involve psychosis, extreme loss of judgment, bankruptcy, impulsivity, and destructive tendencies.

A. When mania occurs, it is highly likely to be followed by additional manic episodes, alternating with depressions, in a condition called bipolar disorder, or manic-depressive illness.

B. The prevalence of bipolar disorder is lower than that of depression—around 2% of the population experiences this condition, roughly evenly divided between men and women.

C. The suicide rate in bipolar disorder is incredibly high— 50% attempt suicide, and untreated, 20% complete suicide, without treatment.

D. Although nearly all forms of mental illness are associated with lowered social class, as either a risk factor or consequence, bipolar disorder is associated, at least in its early phases, with increased productivity and creativity.

E. The heritability of bipolar disorder is far higher than that of unipolar depression, around 80%. Multiple genes are likely to be involved, involving biological rhythms and instability of key neurotransmitter systems.

F. Particularly important for mania is heightened reward sensitivity; people have difficulty in stopping their pursuit of ever-higher goals and rewards.

G. For bipolar disorder, mood stabilizing medication are helpful in reducing manic symptoms and, if taken regularly, in decreasing the risk for future episodes. Education for family members, group support, and other psychological treatments are important adjuncts.

H. Prevention is a key goal. When more specific "risk genes" for severe mood disorders are discovered, there may be dire negative consequences related to eliminating all of those at risk: The genes conferring such risk may also add flavor, insight, sensitivity, and high levels of achievement into our minds and bodies.

V. Overall, the consequences of poor emotion regulation are highly impairing mood disorders, placing a premium on the future discovery of better means of recognizing and coping with negative, and overly positive, emotions and mood states.

Suggested Reading:

Jamison, *An Unquiet Mind.*

Keltner, *Born to be Good.*

Solomon, *The Noonday Demon.*

Whybrow, *A Mood Apart.*

Questions to Consider:

1. When does normative grief or loss cross over into major depression, and what are the implications for both evolution and the means of treating either entity?

2. Mania can be associated with creativity and productivity, so perhaps we should not even treat people with bipolar disorder. Is this a defensible statement; why or why not?

Lecture Eighteen—Transcript
Emotion Regulation and Mood Disorders

Today we continue our emphasis on similarities and differences between the normally functioning mind and the mind that has, in one sense or another, lost its way. Our specific area of strength today is the arena of emotion regulation, with the corresponding area of mental problems denoted by mood disorders, specifically depression and bipolar disorder, which are the consequences of having seriously diminished capacities to regulate one's emotions.

At the outset, let's recall the core lesson from Lecture Six: Namely, emotions are not the disorganizing, irrational, lower-than-human forces they are often stereotyped to be; rather, they organize us, and they focus our attention and motivation on key goals. Without emotions, we cannot perform rational, motivated behavior at all. Still, emotions can be primitive; recall the reptilian emotions of rage—fight or flight—dating from hundreds of millions of years ago in evolutionary time. Without some regulation over them, our lives could be quite difficult indeed.

Parallel to the linkage of ordered rational thought and executive functions to schizophrenia from last time, today's theme is that the human capacity for the regulation of mood is inextricably linked to the risk for serious mood disorders. Let's first get clear about some of the important territory we need to cover today. An emotion, first of all, is a relatively discrete event that typically spans just a few seconds. Certain stimuli tend to trigger happiness, surprise, sadness, anger, fear, and disgust, which are some of the core emotional experiences.

Let's take the latter, disgust: Think right now of rancid, spoiled food. You may have begun already to make a puckered mouth and other signs of the classic disgust emotion—which actually mimics the physical expulsion of food—with very little in the way of elaborate thought. Disgust is one of those phenomena where a preference—in this case, a decided lack of preference—requires very little inference. This kind of response tendency is now widely accepted to be a universal human trait, transcending culture, as the research of Paul Ekman showed. Of course, culture may tell us which foods we do find repulsive and which ones might be considered delicacies; that can differ across cultures.

We can measure the beginning, middle, and end of emotion displays in terms of facial expression, self-reported feelings, and psychophysiology; for example, heart rate, blood pressure, etc. Classic emotion displays do not last much longer than 10 seconds or so. As a side note, consider this: Many, if not most, primary emotions, as well as the key what are sometimes called "social" or "self-conscious" emotions—rage, fear, sadness, shame, embarrassment—are negative. It may have been quite adaptive, in our evolutionary history, to have had a negative bias toward a threatening world, and to have developed a greater number of negative than positive core emotions. Caution and quick defensive, or even attacking, responses to threat were probably those that promoted survival; if we are in doubt about safety versus threat, our naturally selected tendencies tell us to react in a kind of default mode with fear, anger, or disgust to possible threats, as only one "false negative" appraisal—in other words, failing to recognize a stimulus that is a true threat—could end it all.

On the other hand, without positive emotion, we couldn't bond with others; we couldn't procreate, be good parents, or explore new environments. Recall the infant's use of the positive experience of security with a caregiver to explore, quite literally, his or her surroundings if securely attached early on in life. We all tend to do so even later in life in positive relationships and in positive experiences. The field, in fact, known as "positive psychology" is pressing us to consider how we may well be "wired for good."

Next, a mood: On the other hand, this is a longer emotional affective tendency than an emotion per se. I could be in a sour mood for several hours, maybe even all day; or you could feel in quite an elated mood for much of the morning after winning a major prize. But don't think that winning that prize, or hitting the lottery, or moving to a warm-weather climate will—despite what most of us would predict—permanently lift our mood. All of us appear to have a kind of "set point," probably a product of our temperament related to positive affect—we're predisposed to this early in life—and we tend to return to it pretty quickly, even after events that we might predict would give us long-lasting happiness or long-lasting sorrow. Studies show that the effects on our moods of either really good or really bad life events are much more short-lived than we would anticipate. In fact, most of us aren't very good at what we call "affective forecasting": predicting how we'll feel sometime down the road. We all tend to believe, for example, that things will be a lot more negative after adverse events than we usually find them to be not too much later.

Back to mood states: They tend to color just about everything we experience during that time; that morning or that day. In the throes of a really sad mood, all of our emotional experiences tend to the low side; our thoughts get to be negative and pessimistic. This is called "state-dependency" in mood; we tend to recall negative life events and forget positive experiences right at those times. If you are prone to such state-dependent mood effects—and all of us are to some extent—you may recall the kind of feeling of "falling off a cliff"; where did my good feeling go? Why am I only recalling bad or inadequate things that I did? When you do this, you might be gaining some empathy for individuals with clinical depression, who tend to have all too frequently such heart-stopping sensations of utterly low self-worth, gloom, hopelessness, and negative thoughts. In such negative mood states, we even react more quickly to being startled by a loud, sudden sound; it's as though our entire nervous system is tainted by the negative mood state, almost literally jangling our nerves.

A positive mood, in contrast, colors our thoughts, memories, and future projections toward optimism. But if such positive biases get too strong or too frequent, our judgment could get clouded in the other direction; we might actually take undue risks or pursue rewards to a very great extent. Stay tuned; we'll be talking about this in terms of mania. Indeed, my colleague Sheri Johnson, clinical psychologist at Berkeley, has described quite well that the term we call "mania" is often characterized by an excessive pursuit of goals and motivations, in a vicious cycle of ever-greater efforts and costly, often poorly-judged attempts to reclaim that initial "high mood" accompanying the initial success.

Moving on our continuum to emotion and mood, motion scientists and clinicians discuss an even more pervasive style or tendency called "affective tone" or "affective style." This appears to be a proneness throughout life to perceive and experience the world in characteristic ways. A temperamental style first evident in infancy as irritability, impulsiveness, chronic fussiness may predispose the later adult to the Big Five trait we call "neuroticism"; we see the glass as half empty, we don't handle stress very well, we tend to ruminate repeatedly over things that didn't go well during the day. Other individuals appear to be predisposed, from early ages sometimes, to be optimistic and resilient. But, recall from our lectures on temperament, it's a mistake to think that this concept is 100% biological. Early, inborn patterns interact with life experience—and the process we called "goodness of fit"—to shape these sometimes persistent and chronic styles.

Finally, what is a "mood disorder?" Mood disorders might be thought of as the experience of too many negative emotions for too long, or maybe, on the other hand, too many positive emotions in an over-the-top way, as in mania. But mood disorders contain a lot more than difficult mood regulation per se. They are complex syndromes. They typically involve sleep disturbance, sometimes weight gain or loss, negative ways or sometimes overly positive ways of processing information, very low self-perceptions—or again, sometimes very high self-perceptions—and ultimately, what philosopher Albert Camus termed the only true philosophical question: Is life worth living? Mood disorders last anywhere from weeks to months, or in some cases, years at a time; they can involve tremendous heartbreak, impairment, and even disaster.

Let's discuss the 2 major disorders of mood: major depression and bipolar disorder or manic-depressive illness. Let's start with depression. This is a term with multiple meanings; we really need to be careful which of these meanings we're referring to. The term "depression" can signify sad or pessimistic mood; we might call that "small-d" depression. Just about everyone in the world experiences "small-d" depression at one point or another; some are more prone than others. But the term "depression" also refers to a syndrome involving not only sad mood that persists for at least several weeks, but also greatly altered sleep and appetite; extremely low motivation for the things one usually finds pleasurable; self reproach; other characteristic negative thought patterns (for example, all-or-none thinking; over-generalizing from one negative event to everything else; attribution of negative events to what call internal, global, and stable causes, i.e., it's because of me, everything's wrong, and it will always like this); a loss of pleasure is another symptom. In very severe depressions, a person may no longer actually experience sadness, but be almost blank and expressionless.

When depression gets severe enough, the sense is that life is simply not worth living. This syndrome we call "capital-d" depression, or more clinically "major depression"; it's defined officially as at least 2 weeks of these features, experienced nearly every day. A common trigger for many of these symptoms of depression is the experience of a major loss: The death of a loved one, the ending of a deep relationship, or more symbolic losses—terrible failure experiences—typically lead just about all of us to a depressed, withdrawn state for some time. It makes some sense, in terms of evolution, that we humans would shut down, conserve resources, send out emotional signals of distress, and the need for support and nurturance following this kind of major loss. This kind of forced regrouping could give us time to weigh for whom, and how much, we should attach to others in the future. Grieving or bereavement actually includes just about all of the symptoms of major depression I mentioned, except typically there isn't suicidal thinking or excessive guilt.

Here's a clinical question: When does bereavement leave off after a major loss and the signs of a major depression begin? There's really no perfect answer to this question; they're on a spectrum, truly. But if someone is still in the throes of serious grieving half a year or a year later, we might begin to suspect that a tendency toward major depression could underlie the bereavement.

Here's an important fact: Episodes of depression in an individual, except for those directly triggered by a loss that remit pretty quickly, tend to recur; and we call this condition "unipolar depression." Once one has had a major depressive episode, there is actually more than a 50% chance that additional episodes will happen again during the lifetime; so once a severe inability to regulate negative affect takes place, the odds are that it will happen again. Indeed, once one has had 2 depressions, the odds are now 70% or even higher that there will be a third or fourth.

Regarding biology: Once a person is depressed, it could be that serotonin and norepinephrine neurotransmitter systems in the brain readjust somehow. Clear evidence now points, in addition, to changes in the hippocampus—that key structure linked to memory consolidation—as linked to depression. More psychologically, perhaps we get prone to view the world as a hostile place and to begin a pattern of coping that involves more of a retreat than an active stance to the world.

Major depression—capital-d depression—is surprisingly prevalent, especially in adolescent girls and women; it's also a source of clear life impairment. Across the lifespan and around the world, as many as 1 woman in 5, 20%, and about half that many men, 10%, will experience at least one episode of major depression. Here's an interesting developmental and gender-related fact: Before age 11, boys and girls are about equally likely to experience major depression; boys actually might be somewhat more likely. But right at the onset of puberty, between about 12 and 16 years of age, girls skyrocket in their risk. In fact, for the rest of the lifespan, females have twice the risk as males. This pattern is, again, universal and cross-cultural.

Why? Girls and women have a somewhat higher heritability for depression than boys and men; about 40% in females, about 29–30% in males. Girls, too, are socialized to be caregivers and worriers. Female hormones are complexly involved in depressive cycles, as well; and, as we discussed back in Lecture Twelve, the strengths of girls during the first decade of life—their empathy, verbal skills, compliance, social abilities—can actually turn into risk factors during the teen years. More women than men attempt suicide, but more men complete suicide because they tend to use more lethal means (guns, weapons, etc.). Here's an important clinical fact: The suicide risk in someone who has experienced a major depression is typically highest when the person is beginning to recover from a depressive episode; now the energy comes back in so the person is motivated and energetic enough to complete and perform the act.

How can we explain depression; what are some underlying models? In psychoanalytic theory—back recalling Lecture Five—the belief is that any psychological symptoms are the results of biological drives in opposition to social rules, triggering anxieties and then defense mechanisms that we develop unconsciously against the expression of the true nature of these conflicts. In this view, depression is actually the turning inward of the anger one feels in response to this major loss (the departed person, the departed ideal). This defense mechanism has a specific name; it's called "introjection," a turning inward of the aggressive feelings. Better to turn the anger regarding that loss inward than to display hostility to the departed person or ideal, which might be viewed as quite socially unacceptable.

In this perspective, treatment involves expressing the real but unacceptable in social terms, and therefore repressed or introjected anger, and the person then eventually gains insight and works through the conflict. In contrast, social learning/cognitive-behavioral models view depression as the result of thought patterns, characteristic beliefs that turn askew. Individuals resort to black versus white, all or none, over-generalized and ruminative thinking, and a preoccupation with failure and loss. In cognitive behavioral therapy, treatment involves the therapist actively challenging these patterns. The patient works on seeing how emotions might follow from certain beliefs, and then tries out new ways of construing himself or herself and the world. This is a very active therapy, based in the present rather than in past conflicts or losses, and the therapist and patient engage in lots of homework to try out the new ways of thinking outside the therapeutic hour.

A theoretical question is this: Is it that the beliefs—these cognitive distortions—actually precede and trigger the depressed mood, or does sad mood emerge and that triggers these negative thinking patterns. It's not entirely clear. We know that depression does elicit a lot of negative thinking, but perhaps in some people there's a core of dormant or latent negative beliefs that don't show up when the person's not depressed but then kick into gear when the depressive mood comes into play.

Strictly behavioral social learning accounts tend to emphasize the low energy and lack of activation of people with severe depression; so treatments focus on the therapist rewarding the person for getting the person active, for getting out and doing things even though all they do is feel like lying in bed, ruminative and miserable.

What about biological models? Here, depression is thought to result from some forms of dysregulation in the serotonin systems in the brain and the norepinephrine systems in the brain. Antidepressant medications like SSRIs—back in Lecture Two we discussed these—help to regulate neurotransmission of the serotonin system. Other antidepressants work on both serotonin and norepinephrine simultaneously; so they tend to block the serotonin transporter, or the norepinephrine transporter, leaving more of these neurotransmitters in the synaptic cleft. At a deeper level, there's new evidence that these medications do something much more fundamental: They work inside the postsynaptic neuron, actually expressing genes in the cell nucleus. Particularly so in the hippocampus, there may be far more profound impacts of these medications than just simply quickly altering levels of key neurotransmitters.

Here's the clearest evidence we have from research on treating major depression: On average, if we combine very good psychological therapy with optimal medications, the outcome is better than either treatment alone. These are carefully controlled clinical trial research studies, and they support this finding very clearly: Combinations of medication and psychotherapy really enhance the response rates, nearly doubling them in some cases.

Is there a mood state that we might consider the mirror image of depression? What we call "mania" or "manic episodes" is a candidate here. Mania is a mood that begins with expansiveness and elation; ideas are coming alive; the world seems rich with opportunity. Even basic perceptions—sights, sounds, and tastes—are intoxicating. There's a decreased need for sleep; thoughts are sped up. Unlike the withdrawal of depression, life is expansive, and sexual encounters and business ventures tend to multiply. Is this a disorder? Many of us might gravitate towards having these so-called symptoms of the early stages of mania.

But what we call "hypomania"—this first stage that can be quite intensely pleasant—typically progresses to a much darker place. How do we know this? In 1973, psychiatrists Gaye Carlson and Frederic Goodwin published a study called, "The Stages of Mania." They observed patients without medication treatment on a hospital ward with very intense nurse observations, and found that in most cases, this early stage of hypomania progresses into much more serious, advanced stages—they call them stage 2 and 3—they literally kind of take over the person. Let's think: These are not discontinuous stages like Piaget's stages of cognitive development, they're rather phases of a spiraling, unfolding process.

After hypomania, in Stage 2, judgment becomes quite poor; impulse control often gets lost; credit debt; bankruptcy; being fired from jobs; speeding tickets; are typical outcomes. Friends and contacts just can't keep up; the consequences of drug use or unwise sexual encounters can multiply. By the end of Stage 2 of mania, the personal typically becomes psychotic, with hallucinations and delusions that sort of feed the manic/euphoric energy. Hallucinations might involve voices singing the praises of the individual in question. Delusions can be grandiose, with visions of oneself as all-powerful. In an unquiet mind, per her autobiography, Kay Redfield described in one instance how she became preoccupied during a manic episode with penguins, when reading Penguin paperbacks in a bookstore. She then made huge purchases of these books in a misguided manic attempt to save the world's penguins. Irrationality and the beginnings of delusional thinking had clearly taken over by this point.

An important clinical fact: Intense irritability tends to take over from the initial elation. The world isn't keeping up with my grand plans; what's wrong with everyone? Why don't they eagerly respond to my 2:00 a.m. phone calls related to my great business schemes? Again, sexual acting out, substance abuse, and even heart attacks can ensue given the self-absorbed, hyper-energetic, impulsive and irrational symptom picture. At this stage, the risk of suicide gets quite high because the elation can give way to despair, and impulse control gets lost.

In the final stage of mania, called Stage 3, the person is so relentlessly psychotic that he or she is truly indistinguishable from a person with active schizophrenia; the disorganization is now almost total. If a person's had a manic episode, there's a 90% chance that later in life there will be either additional manic episodes, additional depressions, or both; and this is what we call "bipolar disorder," the newer term for what we used to call "manic depressive illness." In this condition, the depressions on average tend to be flat, energy-less, and debilitating. In some individuals, we can plot their life course like clockwork: There are cases of seasonal mood disorder, with summer manias and winter depressions that are quite regular. More typically, however, we can't really predict in an individual at risk for bipolar disorder when the next depression or next mania will occur; or when what we call "mixed states," simultaneous combinations of manic and depressed will ensue.

In fact, mixed states are very problematic. Here the individual might have the negativity, depressed mood, and suicidality of depression, but the energy, drive, and impulsivity of mania, making for a truly lethal combination. I mean lethal, as the risk for suicide is very high at these times.

Across the world, the prevalence of bipolar disorder is a lot lower than that of uni-polar depression; maybe 2% of the world's population experiences some form of bipolar illness, about 50/50 between men and women. Intriguingly, bipolar disorder is the only major form of mental illness that tends to be associated overall with higher, not lower, social class. Initial phases of mania are linked to energy, productivity, creativity; a disproportionate number of poets, sculptors, and other artists tend to have bipolar disorder, unlike a control group of equally prominent biographers, for example. But the destructiveness of later phases of mania typically outweighs this initial creative boost or burst.

I've noted but want to repeat: The suicide rate in bipolar disorder is incredibly high. Without treatment, 50% of people with this condition will make a serious suicide attempt, and about 1 in 5, 20%, will make a suicide attempt that is completed, and they will die. The risk for suicide, as I just mentioned, is particularly high during these "mixed" episodes, where the energy of mania co-occurs with despairing mood; in depressions, too, despair and self-recrimination can predict a loss of hope and suicidality. People with bipolar disorder are at high risk for substance abuse, either to fuel the manias or reclaim that expansive mood when depressions hit hard, or to ease some of that mental anguish of mixed states. In sum, the consequences of unchecked, unregulated mood can be devastating.

What's the heritability of bipolar disorder? It's very high, about 80%. Remember, depression is 30% men, 40% women; bipolar disorder has almost an extreme genetic set of underpinnings. Multiple genes are likely to be involved; these involve not just moods, but biological rhythms and maybe instability of key neurotransmitter systems. But, the relatives of people with bipolar disorder on average tend to be academic, entrepreneurial, and artistic successes. There may be a real advantage to having some partial genetic loading for this condition; and we'll return to this topic in full force in Lecture Twenty-One.

How do we treat this condition? We can't cure it yet, but real, strong, effective treatments do exist. First, mood-stabilizing medications—lithium, plus a host of newer generation medications, even some atypical antipsychotic medicines—can reduce manic symptoms, and if taken regularly, help prevent the risk of later manias and depression. But noncompliance with medication is a big clinical issue; people tend to miss their manic highs, and don't want to be reminded that they have a genetic biochemical disorder. The best psychobiological imitator of a hypo-manic state is what? A cocaine rush. Dopamine systems are amped up completely. People with mania tend to keep seeking ever greater but ever more elusive rewards.

Above and beyond medication, education for family members, group support to motivate the continued taking of medication with peers providing that support motivation; other psychological treatments are very important adjuncts. Serious cases of bipolar disorder almost inevitably require medication; but without insight, and without motivation to stay in treatment and support from therapists, peers, and family members, medication might not ever be taken regularly.

Could we prevent bipolar disorder? It would be a good idea, given how serious its consequences are. But here's a troubling thought: As we come in the future to understand more and more specific risk genes for severe mood disorders, and especially bipolar disorder; we could be getting ourselves into real hot water as a species if we say, "Ah, there's high risk, we should abort that fetus at risk for bipolar disorder." Why? The genes conferring risk for bipolar disorder might also add flavor, insight, sensitivity, creativity, and high achievement to the lives of many individuals. It will really be a challenge for us as a society to come up with preventive measures, given the high lethality of this condition, blended with not only compassion but also our own survival as a species. It would be a grave mistake to cut out the very genes that may make our minds sparkle, or throb with sensitivity—as we see in some phases of depression—if we go too far too fast in terms of the ultimate forms of prevention.

Today's lecture overall has emphasized the following: Mood disorders are quite serious, and they reveal the huge destructive potential that can be unleashed when moods cannot be regulated. On the other hand, depression can foster sensitivity and self-appraisal that's accurate; manic moods in their earliest phases can foster productivity and drive. But all too often, the consequences are devastating, even lethal, when emotion dysregulation is not checked. One of our key challenges is to develop the means of emotion regulation—distancing, reappraising—and applying them in between mood episodes to prevent the full fury of depressions and manias. In most instances, it's going to take medication plus very hard work in psychotherapy and a lot of social support.

Our preventive efforts could backfire, once again, if we strip the human gene pool of those tendencies toward sensitivity and drive. How to prevent serious mood disorders without taking away a key source of human diversity and human strength is sure to be a major scientific, clinical, and ethical issue in the years ahead. Mood disorders are real, often devastating in their consequences, but their roots lie in the emotional and mood-related fluctuations that we all experience.

Lecture Nineteen
Attention, Impulse Control, and ADHD

Scope:

Attention is the filter through which our minds focus on the most salient events inside and around us; inhibitory control allows us to escape previous conditioning and buy time to choose different responses. When attention and inhibition don't function optimally, the controversial diagnosis of attention-deficit/ hyperactivity disorder (ADHD) may result. This lecture reviews the clinical disorder, the impairments related to this condition, as well as medication and behavioral treatments. We will also discuss the ways in which attention and inhibitory disorders can inform us about the normative regulation of attention and behavior.

Outline

I.   Attention is a mental spotlight on the many internal and external stimuli competing for your interest. Inhibitory control allows us to stop previously rewarded responses and choose new plans of action.

   A. There are several types of attention.

   1. Automatic attention occurs when we are unconsciously attracted to a salient stimulus, which may facilitate fight-or-flight responses.

   2. Selective attention pertains to situations in which we choose between competing stimuli (listening to the lecture or thinking of dinner).

   3. Sustained attention is the ability to maintain focus for long periods, despite the tendency to fade and become distracted.

   4. Executive attention is the intentional mustering of energy and cognitive resources to perform difficult tasks.

   5. Attentional capacity/load is related to just how much information we must hold in mind at a given time.

B. Inhibitory control is necessary to delay our response to a stimulus, allowing one to evaluate what to do and plan for alternative courses of action.

II. Evolution clearly favored the ability for individuals to select the most "pressing" situation at hand and devote cognitive resources to it.

A. Across human evolution, an advantage would exist when some individuals tend to display excellent focus and a deliberative cognitive style whereas others display quicker abilities to scan the environment and/or multitask..

B. Genes that are related to attention, focus, and sensation seeking have several alleles, some of which promote greater focus and others of which are associated with a more impulsive style.

C. In contemporary society, however, especially with the advent of compulsory education in the past 150 years, poor focus is a real liability.

III. In modern society, it has long been recognized that high levels of inattention, impulsivity, and hyperactivity are maladaptive.

A. The terms for clinical conditions related to poor focus have shifted from moral defects to minimal brain dysfunction (MBD), hyperactivity, hyperkinesis, ADD, and most recently, attention-deficit/hyperactivity disorder (ADHD).

B. Diagnosis requires extremely high levels of these features, from an early age, in multiple situations, unrelated to recent stress. Prevalence is 6–8% of the school-aged population, which is similar in most nations with compulsory education.

C. As with all other early-onset conditions, boys outnumber girls, by about 3:1.

D. Two main types exist: youth or adults with predominant inattention, and those who display hyperactivity/impulsivity as well.

E. ADHD persists into adolescence and adulthood in a majority of cases. There are high rates of associated aggression, anxiety, learning problems, and, by adolescence, substance abuse and delinquency. For girls, eating problems and depression are common.

IV. ADHD is strongly heritable and is related to other biological risk factors.

    A. The heritability for this condition is 70–80%; higher than that for schizophrenia or depression and comparable to that for bipolar disorder.

    B. As for psychosocial factors, there is little evidence that parenting per se is a causal factor, and there are no elevations of insecure attachment in infants who later develop ADHD. Still, disruptions in parenting and home life may result from having a child with ADHD, and negative, harsh, or lax parenting may well exacerbate the condition.

    C. Reciprocal, transactional models are clearly operative: A child with difficult temperament elicits negative responses from parents, fueling symptoms and related problems. Given ADHD's heritability, it's not uncommon for biological parents to have the syndrome themselves, whether or not diagnosed.

V. Treatments include stimulant medications and behavioral strategies implemented at home and at school.

    A. Why would a child or adult with ADHD respond to a stimulant? It was once thought that the response was paradoxical, but it is now known that all humans respond to low doses of stimulants, which are dopamine agonists, with increased focus.

    B. Over time, however, there can be risk for addiction in adolescents and adults, so stimulants need close monitoring. Considerable debate is occurring over the use of many medications as performance enhancers for the body or mind.

    C. Medication treatment for ADHD is quite effective for most individuals, but effects are short-lived and the optimal results occur when medications are combined with reward-based behavioral programs implemented at home and school.

    D. When medications and behavioral treatments are combined, children who show the largest gains are those whose parents have changed their parenting strategies toward an authoritative style—less harshness, greater consistency.

Suggested Reading:

Barkley, *Attention Deficit Hyperactivity Disorder*.

Hinshaw, *Attention Deficits and Hyperactivity in Children*.

Mayes, Bagwell, and Erkulwater, *Medicating Children*.

Questions to Consider:

1. What are the key advantages and disadvantages of having an attention system that is quick to shift directions, marked by impulsivity and distractibility? Is this a disability or a potential strength?

2. Given that ADHD is not solely an American phenomenon, why is medication use for this condition so much higher in the United States than elsewhere?

Lecture Nineteen—Transcript
Attention, Impulse Control, and ADHD

In the last 2 lectures, we learned that when normative processes of rational thought and executive functions go awry, schizophrenia may result; and when an individual has major problems with emotion regulation, depression or mania may well be the consequences. Today, we feature the mental processes of attention and inhibitory control, and discuss what may transpire when they cannot be performed to their fullest extent. Without attention, the directing of our mental resources toward a specific stimulus, either outside the world or inside our mind, we can be at the mercy of the countless stimuli that impinge on us, many times each and every minute. Without the ability to modulate our own impulses, we are at the mercy of whatever behaviors have been reinforced in the past; so our habits take over, and sometimes these habits are not for the best.

Today our focus is on attention and inhibitory control, and the main condition that can result from deficits in these regulatory systems known as attention-deficit/hyperactivity disorder, or ADHD. Let's start with attention, a key facet of the human mind. Overall, we can think of it as a kind of flashlight or spotlight: Where do we place our mental energies and cognitive resources amidst the sights and sounds, thoughts, memories, feelings, and experiences that surround us every waking moment? In another metaphor, attention is a kind of filter, sifting through these large numbers of stimuli, internal and external, that vie for our interest. Each of our minds actually pays several different kinds of attention. Number 1, some attention is automatic: When we experience a new stimulus, such as flash of light or sound, we orient quickly toward it without any conscious effort, so that our body knows what to do next; whether to flee, fight, or engage.

Number 2, another form of attention involves a kind of choice, and we call this selective attention. As children, for example, do we pay attention to our mother's voice, commanding us to come to dinner, or to the voice of our friend, beseeching us to stay and play? As teens or adults, do we focus on the work at our desk, the text message awaiting us, or the music streaming through our iPod? Research has shown that you can't, in any given exact moment, pay full attention to or more things in the environment, no matter how good a multi-tasker you think you might be; multi-taskers are actually fast switchers.

In fact, can one really multitask well and learn? Let's take a moment here to review some recent research: Some multitasking may, in fact, not be too problematic—listening to music while working, for example—it's just that you're not paying complete attention to the music (or, perhaps, to your work). If each task requires really close attention—texting while doing homework and checking email—there may be more of a problem. Fascinating research from UCLA has shown that when people are asked to track sound tones while at the same time remembering word lists, their initial learning of the word list is not really compromised. But it's when these people are later asked to recall the words; problems emerge then, compared to people who learned the words without having to multitask. The learning while multitasking isn't as deep and retention isn't as strong; in short, it's quite hard to use what you've learned if your learning is done while actively multitasking. Our minds were created to do many things with utter speed and power, but taking in new information—when we do this—the "window" in our minds is actually pretty small and narrow.

Back to attention: After automatic and selective, a third form we call sustained attention. We all experience difficulties with this, when the lecturer drones on and on in a monotone voice, and the chairs are hard, and the material increasingly boring—I really hope you don't lapse in your sustained attention during the next 25 or so minutes. A predominant theory of ADHD has been that people with this condition have real problems with sustaining their attention. We all get drowsy when having to do long, repetitious tasks or listen to monotonous material over and over; but individuals with ADHD, according to this view, have a sharper drop-off than the rest of us. However, other forms of attention—and, perhaps, problems in inhibitory control, which we'll be discussing—may actually be just as salient for ADHD. In other words, some research now shows that people with this condition may have problems with their attention right from the beginning of learning new material, not just a sustained attention drop-off over time.

A fourth form of attention we call executive; recall this concept from our lecture on temperament back in Lecture Eight. We termed this in infancy effortful control. This is the intentional mustering of energy and cognitive resources to concentrate on tasks that are difficult but that may pay off in terms of problem solving later on, if only we can stay focused and engaged. It is this form of attention that involves not just focus, but a number of executive functions like planning, maintaining our orientation despite distractions, and coping with errors that may really well be the core of ADHD.

Number 5, we can think of attention, in addition, as having a size, capacity, or load. How many numbers can you recall of this list that I read randomly one per second? 2 … 7 … 3 … 1 … 8 … 4 … 5 … 9. We sometimes call this a kind of working memory, but it does require careful attention to recall more than the average for most adults, which is about 7 bits of such information. Here's a new series of numbers; please repeat them after I'm done in backwards order: 7 … 1 … 4 … 5 … 2 … 6 … 9 … 3. This much more difficult task requires not only attention and memory, but also some executive skills, like grouping or chunking units together. Before we stored phone numbers in computers or cell phones, this was the way, for example, to remember long-distance phone numbers of 10 digits: 3 for the area code, 3 for the prefix, and 4 for the rest of the number. Each of these types of attention engages different regions and different circuits of the brain. It would take the entire lecture to go through all of the relevant neuroanatomy, but the point for now is that attention is not just one thing, either in terms of what it does or its underlying brain capacity.

What's the optimal attentional style to strive for? Across evolution, we can envision a selective advantage when some individuals would display very strict focus and a deliberative cognitive style, with high levels of executive attention. Indeed, this is what we humans supposedly do so much better than other species. But in certain human environments, other individuals may have had quicker abilities to scan the environment, a kind of multitasking, or at least fast-tasking. Diversity in a population tends to produce reproductive advantage as environments and settings change.

Here's a provocative finding: There are some genes that are related to our abilities to pay attention and focus—or, on the other hand, to be prone to sensation seeking; taking risks, being more exploratory—and these genes often have 2 or more alleles. Here's an example of the DRD4 gene—the dopamine receptor type-4 gene—that essentially instructs the body to produce more of the fourth type of receptor for dopamine in the brain. One allele of this gene actually produces lower levers of this receptor; it's known as the 7-repeat allele, because a particular sequence of base pairs repeats 7 times. This allele is linked to sensation-seeking in the population, and, as we'll soon describe, to the condition we call ADHD. Geneticists have determined that this allele existed in relatively low frequencies around 15,000 years ago in Asian populations. But then, as the latest Ice Age receded—there was an actual land mass across what is today the Bering Strait—some humans with the sensation-seeking form of this gene (the 7-repeat allele) were those who were more likely to explore and cross the Strait into the western part of the New World. There are higher frequencies of this 7-repeat allele among the descendants of those who made the migration than among those who stayed behind. The frequencies get ever higher the further down the coast of current Canada, the United States, and beyond we go.

Here's a great example of natural selection at work: As environmental change "pushed" for new and adaptive behaviors, genes linked to certain traits—in this case exploration—actually increased in frequency, given the reproductive advantages they'd produced. This is, indeed, natural selection at work. In this case, natural selection's products—higher frequencies of this genotype—show expansion not only over time, but across regions of the world. There appears to have been selection pressure for, in some cases, a more exploratory style; more of that style ended up in the Americas than in Asia. But let's fast forward now to modern society: With the advent of compulsory education over the last 150 years, poor focus—maybe a link to sensation-seeking—is a real liability; it can make for major problems with school. With 500 or more channels today, with the Internet, instant messaging, and the like, what is the most adaptive attentional style? Could contemporary culture actually be driving all of us to become less attentive? These are provocative questions, and we don't yet have the full answers.

Beyond attention, another essential function of our minds is the ability to delay responding to a stimulus in the environment, especially one that has previously been linked with to a behavior producing a reward, and to evaluate just what we want to do. This skill is called inhibition or inhibitory control. It is linked to impulse control; or, if we word it in the other direction, impulsivity. The idea is this: Sometimes we are victims of habit, even folly, if we always respond without a chance to really think what we want to do. Using more technical terms, we often show a "prepotent" response to a previously rewarded stimulus.

Think of social learning theory and operant conditioning: Once a reward schedule has been maintained, we tend to respond similarly when a stimulus comes up in our environment. But it really may help to think for a moment what you really want to do in a given situation. You're now a child in a classroom, and you're briefly recalling the thrill last week of the other kids' laughter when you shot that perfectly spherical spitball toward the teacher's desk. But now, can you restrain yourself from the impulse to do so again—even though that act was rewarded last week—especially as you now realize the teacher has promised you'll be sent home or even suspended if you do it once more? Those crucial milliseconds after a stimulus—in this case, recalling how it felt last week—really defines where the action is; will you impulsively respond as you did last time, or can you stifle or inhibit that prepotent response and use your executive functions to decide on what you really want to do? There are different types of inhibition, just as there were with attention, such as inhibiting certain behaviors when we're fearful, or inhibiting behavior when we have a higher-order goal in mind. But they share the element of interrupting an ongoing, previously rewarded stream of behavior.

A prominent theory of ADHD, from psychologist Russell Barkley, is that this condition does not really constitute a fundamental problem of attention nearly as much as it's a fundamental problem of inhibitory control. If we have problems with this core function, if we have poor inhibitory control, we cannot even get our executive functions kicked into gear to plan and monitor our behavior, because we're victims of our past learning and behavior, over and over.

In modern society, then, what are the consequences when an individual has extremes of inattention, very poor inhibitory control, and possibly high levels of fidgeting, squirminess, and hyperactivity? The terms for clinical conditions linked to such problems have shifted over the years; they were called, actually, "moral defects" at the turn of the 20th century—note here the clear juxtaposition of a naturalistic model with a social deviance or moral view—then later minimal brain dysfunction, hyperactivity, hyperkinesis, ADD (attention-deficit disorder), and now most recently, ADHD (attention-deficit/hyperactivity disorder). We should diagnosis this condition only when an individual shows very high levels of these features, compared to others of the same sex or same age; a statistical model is often used for initial diagnosis. We should insist that the problems are present from an early age in multiple situations in home and school, or home and the workplace, and unrelated to recent stress; then, and only then, should we consider

©2010 The Teaching Company.

a diagnosis. Around 6, 7, or 8% of the school-aged population received such a diagnosis; this is a very similar rate across all nations that have compulsory education. But there may be higher proportions of individuals with, for example, the 7-repeat allele of the DRD4 gene in certain venues such as North America than in other regions.

Like all other early-onset behavioral and emotional conditions of childhood—autism, aggression, some forms of learning disorders—that tend to begin before the age of 10, boys outnumber girls, and for ADHD this is about 3:1. This leads to an intriguing sidelight: Why are boys truly at greater risk for the behavioral disorders of childhood than girls? This could take us far from today's topic, but one brief answer is that the Y chromosome—which confers and triggers maleness, as we've discussed—is actually quite physically small compared to the X chromosome; it has very few genes on it. In an XY individual, a genetic male, it may protect against any genetic vulnerability in the corresponding X chromosome; indeed, boys are more vulnerable than girls to a whole host of genetic and environmental risk factors early in life.

Back to ADHD, there are 2 main forms: Some youth display predominant problems in inattention, disorganization, and lack of focus; we call them the inattentive type, it used to be called ADD without hyperactivity in the 1980s. Others display lots of hyperactive/impulsive behavior, or what we just called poor inhibitory control, in addition to the inattention. We call such individuals the combined type, meaning that they have a combination of both types of symptoms. These are the stereotypic kids with ADHD; however, the inattentive type, although not as disruptive, often has major problems with school, motivation, and with later life success. For the record, there is a purely hyperactive-impulsive type, too; this is usually confined to preschool or kindergarten children. Their inattentiveness doesn't really show up until first grade or beyond with the demands of formal schooling.

The majority of time, a person validly diagnosed with ADHD persists with these symptoms and problems into adolescence, and even into adulthood half the time. The extremes of overactivity and fidgetiness could recede by adolescence, but the underlying attention problems and inhibitory control deficits do tend to persist.

When a person meets criteria for ADHD, there's a strong likelihood that aggressive behavior and learning problems may develop, and anxiety can ensue; and by adolescence, there's a high risk for substance abuse and, in some cases, delinquency. In girls with this condition, eating problems and depression are common; having major problems with regulation of attention and major problems with inhibitory control tend to pave the way for other, impairing mental problems. This is really a sign of how crucial attentional capacities and inhibitory control are for our lives in this present era. Girls can and do get ADHD, and when they have it, the consequences may even be more severe than they are for boys.

Let's review some of the impairments: Boys and girls with ADHD are highly likely to have problems in school and achievement, even if they don't have formal learning disabilities. Next, children with ADHD tend to be more disliked than children with any other mental condition. Think of this: The child with ADHD is too often the one to blow out the candles at that birthday party, even though it's not his or her birthday, it's the other kids'. Kids don't like that impulse control, and we now know that with the importance of peer rejection, kids with ADHD maintain difficult consequences later in life.

Third, families get disrupted; there are arguments, tears over homework, and defiance. Fourth, and quite tellingly, accidental injury related to impulsive, risk-taking behavior is occurring at high rates in individuals with ADHD. During preschool, high rates of accidental injury; after the age of 16, 17, or 18, individuals with this condition are at high risk for serious accidents in cars. They are real health impairments. This is really in opposition to the media stereotypes we see in some cases, claiming that we tend to label difficult, nonconforming behavior as disordered because of social control. In fact, ADHD does yield high risk for key developmental problems across the lifespan.

What might cause inattention and impulse control to get into the ADHD range? First, ADHD is quite heritable; the heritability is 70–80%. This is higher than the statistic we talked about 2 lectures ago for schizophrenia and last time for depression; it's comparable to the 80% for bipolar disorder. Even though our main stereotype is that ADHD is just the result of lax or permissive parenting, genes play a major role in contributing to the risk for ADHD and individual differences in these symptoms.

There are multiple genes involved: those related to dopamine, like the DRD4 gene we've just been talking about, but undoubtedly many others. Here's an intriguing finding from the last few years: In longitudinal research using brain imaging, in children with ADHD, the expected thinning of the cortex during middle to late childhood was delayed by about 3 years in contrast to normally developing youth. During the crucial years of childhood, there appear to be differences in brain maturation processes linked to ADHD. This finding indeed mirrors the clinical observation that many kids with ADHD appear to be immature in their behaviors and their emotion regulation capacities. The developmental timing of brain functions could be a major role in certain developmental disorders like ADHD.

There are other potential causes, too: if you're born at low birth weight; if your mother drank or smoked during pregnancy; there's some link to increased behaviors related to ADHD from preschool ingestion of dyes and additives. I could discuss all of these factors at length, but the point is that evidence is accumulating that they could lead to compromises in just those brain regions and circuits that help us regulate our behaviors, and that are responsible for executive and impulse control.

What about psychological factors? There's actually little evidence that parenting styles per se are a causal factor in ADHD. There's actually no increased rate of insecure attachment in infants who later develop ADHD, but insecure attachment in the earliest years is a predictor of later aggressive behavior.

Let's make a simple model here; it's oversimplified, but we might begin to think of ADHD as quite heritable and quite neurocognitive. But some forms of aggression actually have more of a deep attachment-based emotional route; it's more complex than this, but this would give us a basic, rule-of-thumb guideline. In fact, we have to remember the all-important presence of reciprocal and transactional models: Parents may react to the child with a difficult, dysregulated temperament with anger, frustration, and giving up on rule setting; but those kinds of responses from parents are likely to amplify the underlying biological vulnerability and would lead to longer-lasting ADHD or to promote additional aggressive behavior.

Note this: Because ADHD is substantially heritable, it's likely that a third or even more of biological parents of kids with this condition have at least some form of ADHD themselves, or at least they are on the continuum. This is important clinically: Parents of kids with

ADHD really need to be super-attentive, super-regulated, and quite regular with their discipline. This is hard enough for any parent, but it would be especially so if you, as a parent, have impulse control problems yourself.

What's the true cause of ADHD? We have to nominate compulsory education. I say this partly tongue in cheek, but not completely: We didn't really notice children with extremes of inattention and impulsivity before we made them do things for which our minds didn't really evolve (sitting for long hours in seats, learning to read). There are clearly genes and other biological risk factors that make certain children salient in such settings. It's also true that extremes of inattention could have led to problems even in hunter-gatherer or agrarian cultures, but the environments back then were not as demanding of attention and impulse control as they clearly are now.

How do we treat ADHD? Many different interventions have been used over the years, but there are only 2 with a strong evidence base: Number one, the stimulant medications, which are dopamine and norepinephrine reuptake blockers; and then second, behavioral treatments from social learning theory implemented at home and school (regular reward, regular not severe punishments for misbehavior). Neurofeedback or biofeedback (regulating one's own brain waves) is gaining credence as a treatment these days, too. It would seem paradoxical at first: Wait a minute, here's a child or adult with ADHD, they're already "hyper"; why would they respond positively to a stimulant medication? The fact is, though, that nearly all humans show better focus on low doses of stimulants, even the caffeine in coffee. At low to moderate dosage levels, stimulants actually stimulate those dopamine and norepinephrine pathways in the brain needed for attention and inhibitory control. Could we put stimulants in the water supply, the way we do with fluoride, and help everybody be more attentive? The reason we don't, of course, is that stimulants can be addictive for adolescents and adults, and careful monitoring is needed. But there's a lot of interest these days in what we call neuro-enhancement, the use of "steroids of the mind," as stimulants are sometimes referred to, to help everyone's mental and cognitive abilities; it's clearly a hot topic.

Stimulants, like Ritalin and its longer-acting forms and amphetamines in their longer-acting forms present a key issue today: They are performance enhancers, use of which might be desirable for exam studying, late night performance, and the like across the whole population. Their use, and potential abuse, demonstrate that attention and impulse control do exist on a continuum; there do not appear to be any qualitative black-white differences between those with ADHD and those without. The statistical model, the continuum model, may well apply here.

At a clinical level, substantial evidence—hundreds of controlled studies—show that well-delivered and well-monitored medication can be highly beneficial for many kids with ADHD, though again, they are not a cure. Recent studies show that the benefits of these medicines, however, when given for a few years of childhood, don't automatically translate into long-term benefits in adolescence or adulthood. It appears that we really need to sustain treatment for this condition, more like a chronic disorder than a transitory, "infectious" disease. What about non-medication treatments? One-on-one therapy doesn't work terribly well for people with ADHD; on the other hand, behavioral treatments, based, again on social learning theory—regular, consistent rewards at home and school—can be quite effective.

What do we know? When we combine medications and well-delivered behavioral treatments, the gains are the best and strongest. I've been involved myself in a carefully controlled study at Berkeley with my colleagues there and 5 other centers around the United States and Canada in what we call the MTA Study. Here's what we found across the years: To improve the core symptoms of ADHD, but also to reduce aggression and anxiety, and in addition to increase academic performance, social skills, and families' discipline strategies at home, it really does take a combination of well-monitored medication plus intensive behavior therapy at school, at home, and during summer programs with the child. The best reductions in problems and the most improvements in their impairments appear to occur with combination, multimodal treatment.

Our research group at Berkley led a study to show something, to me, even more fascinating: Even though ADHD has a substantial heritability (80%, as we discussed earlier) when children with ADHD received this combination treatment, and, in some cases, when their parents showed pretty darn dramatic improvement in their parenting styles—they became less negative, much more consistent—these children not only improved, but they looked indistinguishable from their non-ADHD classmates at school; their behavior was normalized for the time of treatment.

What's the lesson? Even for conditions with quite strong heritability, like ADHD, changes in the environment—the home environment, more consistent discipline—can still lead to better outcomes; another myth-busting finding related to heritability. Heritability, again, doesn't mean that environments are unimportant for the individual case.

Overall, the human mind and the behaviors that emanate from the mind and in our bodies can be malleable, despite, in some cases, biological, heritable origins that are strong. The more one knows, the harder it is to separate nature from nurture. ADHD, in fact, provides fresh evidence that even strongly heritable mental disorders can respond to changes in the environment as well as to medications, and especially the combination of the 2. Once again, heritability is not destiny.

Lecture Twenty
Empathy, Social Connections, and Autism

Scope:

Social relatedness and empathy are key parts of our evolutionary heritage; extremely poor social skills are likely to yield devastating life consequences. This lecture discusses altruism and the controversial topic of group selection; theory of mind, the mental module, emerging during the preschool years; and autism, the condition in which children show social isolation, language abnormalities, and highly restricted interests from the first years of life. The autism "epidemic," distinctions from Asperger's disorder, the high heritability of this condition, and the effects of early behavioral interventions are also covered.

Outline

I. Social connections and empathy are foundations of humanity.

    A. In human evolution, our species couldn't have survived and reproduced without a strong penchant for social behavior.

    B. Empathy can be divided into emotional empathy, taking on the feelings of others, and cognitive empathy, understanding those feelings in others.

II. Between 3 and 5 years of age, humans develop theory of mind, the ability to understand that other people may have different perspectives than oneself.

    A. Even children with mental retardation "pass" theory of mind tests at the correct chronological or developmental age.

    B. But if you couldn't develop this ability, or could only do so through laborious mental efforts, the social world would be a confusing place, indeed. This may well be a core deficit of the condition we call autism, as even high-functioning individuals with autism fail theory of mind tasks.

    C. Evolutionary psychologists posit that theory of mind is a discrete mental module, but others contend that it may emerge from relationship quality as well.

III. Autism was discovered in the 1930s and 1940s as a disorder beginning in the earliest years of life, involving 3 core deficits.

   A. Language problems and delays: Some autistic individuals never learn to speak, whereas others have language oddities, such as repeating precisely what's just been said, or extremely focused conversations about restricted topics.

   B. Social isolation and difficulty bonding with others: Parents report that, during the first months of life, many children with autism recoil from being held. Eye contact is poor, and many youth with autism appear to use others as objects rather than real people.

   C. Repetitive play and need for preservation of sameness: Autism is marked by extremes of behavioral rigidity, with some children throwing violent tantrums to any alteration in schedule or routine.

   D. Whereas most youth with autism function intellectually in the mentally retarded range, a subgroup has "high functioning autism," with good language skills. This group is sometimes defined as having Asperger's disorder.

   E. Case studies exist where autistic savants have incredible memory, musical, or mathematical calculation abilities. Despite media popularization, such individuals appear to be relatively rare.

   F. Longitudinal studies reveal that autism is rarely outgrown, although some individuals with high-functioning autism can lead semi-independent lives.

IV. Claims abound that autism is skyrocketing in prevalence. Data from the past 10 years indicate that rates have tripled in some venues.

   A. Is there a true increase in prevalence? This is highly unlikely. Rather, a spectrum of autism and other pervasive developmental disorders are now diagnosed far more than ever before, because of the visibility of the condition and its established nature in helping to procure special school services.

B. One provocative idea is the Silicon Valley Syndrome, whereby 2 parents, each with well developed mathematical and spatial abilities but rather poor social skills, mate and produce offspring with heightened genetic risk.

V. What are the causes of this mysterious condition?

   A. Heritability is as high as that for any psychiatric condition, as high as 90%. There may be other biological risk factors, in utereo, that accentuate or potentiate the genetic risk.

   B. Contrary to original views that faulty parenting produced autistic reactions in children, in many cases the symptoms are present in the earliest months of life; many children with autism actually show secure attachment; and a quarter of children with autism will develop seizures by adolescence or early adulthood, clearly signifying neurological rather than psychological roots.

   C. A subset of children with autism appear to develop normally during the first year of life but then regress significantly during the second year. For them, head circumferences may be overly large, possibly signifying that an underlying mechanism is a failure in neural pruning—leading to large but inefficient brains.

   D. As noted above, even high-functioning children with autism do not "pass" theory of mind tests by age 5, signifying that autism may relate to a specific deficit in perspective taking.

VI. The most documented intervention strategy for autism is intensive, in-home behavioral interventions emphasizing rewards and skill-building, for at least 20 hours per week, during the preschool years. Although initial claims that such treatment would cure autism in 50% of cases were overstated, early stimulation, training, and rewards can help establish language, cognitive, and behavioral skills that may allow for regular education.

Suggested Reading:

Grandin, *Thinking in Pictures*.

Offit, *Autism's False Prophets*.

Sigman and L. Capps, *Children with Autism*.

Questions to Consider:

1. Why does it make psychological and evolutionary sense that some of us are gregarious whereas others are far more socially withdrawn isolated?

2. At what point on the continuum of social relatedness and linguistic ability should we consider diagnosing an individual with a condition like autism—in other words, how stringent should the diagnostic threshold be?

Lecture Twenty—Transcript
Empathy, Social Connections, and Autism

Today, we conclude our set of lectures on crucial strengths of the human mind and what happens when we they don't fully develop. Our focus today is on the absolutely critical functions of social connectedness and empathy; without these we couldn't have survived as a species beyond a few short generations. The condition that results from fundamental problems in these mechanisms is called autism, which typically appears during the first 2 years of life. There's already a fundamental insight here: A disorder that is, at its core, a disruption in social relatedness begins to show itself during the initial months of human existence. This is core evidence that without social bonds, we are at risk of becoming quite impaired just as our minds are actively forming.

Autism is the source of much fundraising today, much research, and much controversy, related to its prevalence, as well as its causes and treatments. We'll deal with some of that controversy; but let's get oriented first to the facets of the normally developing mind that could get sidetracked in individuals with autism.

Today's focus is on sociability, interpersonal connections, and empathy, those necessary tools for life as humans; and on what can go terribly wrong when such basic socioemotional skills and processes don't develop in timely fashion. As has been the case so often in this course, let's begin with evolutionary principles. With our species—which lacks the size and strength to compete with key predators; and which requires long periods of helplessness, in order for the development of our plastic brains and minds—there was strong selection pressure for the following: forming close, lasting relationships with others, both clans and tribes; and attaching to intimate partners, and to our children. In other words, in the evolution of our species, we couldn't have survived and reproduced without a strong drive for social behavior. It's quite clear, then, that natural selection favored those humans who desired social contact.

We're not alone in this orientation; many mammalian and especially primate species are quite social. But we have developed sophisticated ways of relating to others, especially given how much we depend on our fellow humans to transmit culture and innovation, and especially given how long we stay helpless when we're young. But negotiating a social group is no picnic; think of your colleagues at work, or think of family reunions. Dating and courting are no easy matters, either. What about the intricacies of parenting: that combination of giving, providing, nurturing, scaffolding, and limit-setting, and then gradually letting go as the child develops? It takes real skill to understand the social motives of our fellow humans, and to predict and respond to the emotions of others.

But note—in a point that will become much clearer in Lecture wenty-Two—we humans could not have evolved an indiscriminate, "all-purpose" social drive. To avoid contagion or exploitation, humans also had to have some "brakes" on our social contacts and social bonds; otherwise, an indiscriminately friendly, sociable human would have been literally taken advantage of. What's crucial is the development of an ability to "read" other people, both to be able to bond with them and, at times, to be wary of them. Even more, we sometimes have to hide our own goals and intentions; equally, we have to be quite good at detecting deceit and being cheated from others. This is complicated stuff. The need for these kinds of social and emotional skills is likely to be a key factor, in terms of natural selection, that drove our larger and more connected brains and minds.

A core set of abilities and sensitivities along this line is found in the term empathy. One form is called emotional empathy, literally, experiencing the feelings of others as though they were ours. Early forms of this kind of empathy are apparent even in infancy: 1-month-old babies will mimic the distress cries of other infants that they hear. Developing later, somewhere around 3 years of age, maybe earlier—when the mind is more able to understand that other people have separate, distinct minds—is what we call "cognitive empathy," the understanding of just what feelings another may be experiencing; so it's an understanding, not just a shared feeling.

The relationship between emotional and cognitive empathy is quite intriguing. Pure emotional empathy can be a powerful experience; for example, when we suddenly "get" how someone who has lost a parent, a child, or a life partner really feels. It's almost as though we've been hit over the head, sensing as though it were we who were feeling that pain. But staying in that kind of emotionally attuned place at times can be overwhelming; how can we really understand what they're feeling

©2010 The Teaching Company.

but not be completely caught up in its force? Cognitive empathy comes into play. Indeed, we would probably like our therapists and our closest confidants and friends to be rich in cognitive empathy, understanding our conflicts and painful experiences, but not getting so wrapped up in them that they can't help out.

Prosocial behavior is relevant here; in other words, behavior expressly intended to help or aid someone else. It could result from the emotional and cognitive empathy we've just described; and the task is to understand the negative emotions of others and come to aid the person who is distressed.

Here's a major evolutionary puzzle: Why, in fact, would any individual be empathic at all? Why would an individual work to further the goals, even the survival, of someone else at the expense of his or her own survival? Aren't we all driven by natural selection to favor our own goals and purposes, our own genes, first and foremost? This is a topic of real complexity; it continues to receive scrutiny from evolutionary theorists and research investigators. One solution, expressed by the eminent genetic theorist Richard Dawkins, is that although genes are inherently "selfish," wishing only to reproduce themselves, such selfish genes could yield, in complex organisms, behavior that could be cooperative, even sometimes self-sacrificing.

One venerable evolutionary theory in this regard was termed group selection; perhaps, for the good of the species, some members sacrificed themselves. This view fell out of favor during the latter part of the 20th century among evolutionists. Genes, in fact—it was contended—are "motivated" to reproduce themselves, not to produce behaviors that help others; this came to be the common belief. But noted evolutionary biologists, including E. O. Wilson, the founder of sociobiology and evolutionary psychology, have helped to lead kind of a comeback of the idea of group selection. Although for individuals, selfish behavior is typically the better strategy, for groups as whole, survival may well be ensured by the altruistic behavior of at least some members.

For a complex, social species, and one that could need many hands on deck to evade predators and form bonds and bands, "reciprocal altruism" indeed makes sense. This isn't pure sacrifice, but is a kind of tit-for-tat, or a planned trade or share of goods, services, or helpful behaviors. If I help you today—sharing food, for example—you may well be more likely to help me tomorrow by sharing back in turn.

This was highly likely to have been a complex social behavior shaped by evolution throughout much of human history, when the next meal, dependent on the next hunt, was no certainty at all. But think about this: If I really have reciprocal altruism, I have to be able to time travel, with a vengeance. I have to understand that my action today will have a reasonable chance of being reciprocated by you tomorrow; my survival, after all, depends on it. I have to be quite skilled in my judgment that you will, in fact, reciprocate.

Here's another evolutionary concept called "kin selection," which we'll cover briefly. The idea is that I may well sacrifice myself for the protection and survival of my offspring, my siblings, and any others who share significant genes with me. In fact, we humans are quite attuned—even exquisitely attuned—to patterns of kinship; our social interactions and social cognitions have been shaped by natural selection to recognize and seek information about them, and we are willing, often, to develop highly altruistic behaviors to promote survival of the genes of close kin because in that sense our own genes are propagated.

Parenthetically, I want to mention a discovery made in the late 1990s, the implications of which are still being probed today: mirror neurons. In a number of mammalian species, some neurons in the sensory regions and the motor regions of our parietal lobes respond to seeing someone else reaching, touching, or recoiling just as though we ourselves were reaching, touching, or recoiling. In other words, these neurons literally mirror others' actions as though they were our own actions. This is remarkable; maybe a true neural basis of empathy. It's controversial just how much of a role mirror neurons play in complex human behaviors. Some of the popular stories on these specialized neurons have really outstripped the actual evidence that there is a purely neuronal basis for all empathy in humans. Still, Ramachandran of UC San Diego and others have speculated that autism might relate to mirror neuron problems in this subgroup of human children.

The bottom line is this: It's possible, and, in fact, necessary, to have social bonds and cooperative behavior in balance with more purely self-centered motives. A key building block of human cooperation and social behavior is the understanding that others have perspectives, thoughts, and feelings that really may be separate quite separate from my own. Human infants and toddlers are indeed "wired" to ascribe human qualities, and agency, to a host of inanimate objects. Let's recall some material from an earlier lecture: Between 3 and 5 years of age roughly, what we call theory of mind develops. This is the ability to literally understand that other people have different perspectives than oneself. It's a crucial developmental milestone for the developing child.

Let's be concrete: How do we assess this function? A classic means is called the Smarties test (Smarties are Britain's version of M&Ms). Here's the scenario: The young child is given a Smarties box, but the experimenter comes in and diabolically fills it with pencils. Then, another person enters the room; the first child is asked, "What will she think is in the box?" By about 4 years of age, give or take, the child will say, "Duh, Smarties!" The inner monologue might be something like this: "Well, of course, the other child will think Smarties are in the box; he or she didn't see the Smarties being replaced by pencils, only I did." But younger children will typically say, assuming that their own egocentric view is the only valid one, "pencils." It's hard for very young child to give up his or her fundamental egocentrism. By 3 ½, 4, 4 ½ years of age, children in this view have developed a literal theory of mind, the belief and knowledge that other minds are fundamentally different from one's own.

What's the science tell us? There have been actually been some challenges to this particular way of testing for theory of mind. If we somehow could simplify the many cognitive requirements of the task (a lot of working memory involved), or take away the subject's ability to have to remember all these sequences (a Smarties box, replaced with pencils, other child comes in), theory of mind can be seen even earlier during development, before 3. It may not be that it's quite as dramatic or sudden a "stage" of development as some have thought. But a core view is that theory of mind is akin to a mental module, a kind of innate skill that emerges with pretty minimal environmental input somewhere around 3 ½ or 4; it's a discontinuous stage in development from this perspective.

But other studies reveal that, in fact, the ways that parents socialize their children to understand others and to comprehend others' feelings may also contribute to the development of theory of mind; it's not just the biological emergence of a fully instinctive module. Lots of developmental research is probing and debating these competing ideas.

But here's a really crucial finding: Children with mental retardation—for example, Down's syndrome—can "pass" theory of mind tests (understand the perspective of others) at the correct chronological or in some cases the correct "cognitive" age; some pass it when they're about 3 ½ or 4, or when their mental age comes to that level. They're mentally retarded and don't have full intellectual skills, but they pass theory of mind tasks at the particular age.

But what if you couldn't develop this ability, or what if you could only figure it out through laborious calculations and mental efforts? The social world would be really confusing. Indeed, this is believed by some scientists and clinicians to be the core deficit of the condition we call "autism," because even high-functioning individuals with autism—those of normal intelligence—tend to fail theory of mind tasks well past the age of 4, and even taking into account their mental age. For those people with specific deficits in this ability, social relationships would, again, be quite compromised; the individual in question can't really "relate" to others as separate, autonomous beings with views, feelings, and motivations different from one's own. The consequences, in fact, could be quite devastating.

Let's examine the clinical picture of children and older individuals with autistic disorder, and how this condition potentially links with theory of mind. In the very late 1930s and the early 1940s, Professor Kanner in the United States and Dr. Asperger in Europe independently discovered similar clinical conditions. In both cases, rare groups of children were shown to display severe social deficits, often from the earliest years of life. Kanner called this "early infantile autism," "autism" the term signaling a sense of core isolation. Kanner was the eminent head of child psychiatry at Johns Hopkins University in Baltimore, people flocked around the world to get his opinion; and he defined 3 core symptom areas. First: language problems and delays; indeed, many autistic individuals never learn to speak at all. Others who do speak show language oddities—for example, repeating precisely what's just been said, called echolalia—or they show quite focused conversations about restricted, specialized topics (streetcars, trains, hobbies).

The second symptom area: social isolation and difficulty bonding with others. Indeed, parents report that, during the first months of life, many children with autism recoil from being held. Eye contact with the parent is poor or nonexistent. Some children with autism appear to use others as kinds of objects rather than real people; grabbing an adult's hand to get a toy, not really understanding that this adult is a separate human being with his or her own feelings. There's a process called "joint attention": The child looks to the parent who's pointing and saying, "Look, a kitty," and the child follows that point and gaze. This is a crucial social task in the first few months of life, into the second year of life, but in autism joined attention develops poorly, if at all.

The third area of symptoms involves repetitive play and a real need for the preservation of routine. Autism is, in fact, marked by extremes of very rigid behavior; some children tantrum violently to any alteration, even minute, in schedule or routine. Kanner called this an "obsessive need for preservation of sameness"; it's like a kind of needing the world to be explicitly controllable, any deviation cannot be tolerated. To get a diagnosis of autistic disorder, children have to display very debilitating patterns in these 3 areas during the first 3 years of life; so it's an early-onset condition.

In passing, Asperger, in Europe, saw very bright children and adolescents who did have spoken language, sometimes quite sophisticated; but they typically had specialized, very peculiar interests and would not be able to handle or manage any deviation from those topics. Their language was sometimes stilted, and not very responsive to others. Today we use the term "Asperger's disorder" to refer to youth or adults with what otherwise called "high-functioning autism"; in fact, these 2 diagnoses are almost interchangeable, although some contend that there are subtle differences.

Both are part of what we call "autism-spectrum disorders." Indeed, rather than the view of half a century ago that autism was an extremely rare, uniformly devastating condition, we've shifted in recent years to the view that autism occurs along a spectrum or continuum, just like the other mental disorders we've discussed in this course. Relatively few children have the full autism disorder, with severe problems in communication, social abilities, play, and restricted interest; but a larger number have some degree of difficulty in several if not all of these domains.

What was the initial view about ideology and causation? Kanner and others also thought that emotional refrigeration from parents who simply could not bond with their child was the cause. They also believed—the originators of the concept—that autism was exclusively a white, upper-middle-class or upper-class phenomenon. But this was clearly what we call "referral bias"; in the early days, only quite wealthy families could travel to the few centers in the world that specialized in this mysterious new condition called "autism." Let's think of our many earlier discussions of reciprocal and transactional models: Perhaps some parents react to a child's lack of social bonds with frustration, distance, and a kind of despondency; so the parent's actually responding to the child. Because autism is extremely heritable—about 90% so—biological parents may well have at least some autistic features themselves.

Here's another key point: Most children with autism, around 3/4, function intellectually and cognitively in the mentally retarded range; it could range from mild to severe, again, many children with autism have no spoken language at all. But there's a subgroup, about a quarter, who show what we call "high functioning autism," with good language skills; although, again, somewhat unusual or idiosyncratic language production is salient. Case studies exist where there are a few autistic "savants" who have incredible memory or musical or mathematical abilities; think of the film *Rain Man*, for example. Despite media popularization, such individuals are quite rare.

Crucial for this belief that autism is linked closely to a fundamental deficit in theory of mind is that even high-functioning autistic individuals—with high IQ scores, good intellectual abilities—do not quickly understand and pass theory of mind tests. They might take many more years before they can automatically "get" this; instead, they analytically sort out, "Here's another person, they may have a different perspective than mine." It's laborious, effortful processing, not a quick mental module clicking into gear.

Longitudinal studies show that autism is rarely outgrown; but some high-functioning individuals with autism can, in fact, lead semi-independent lives. In other words, the long-term consequences of a failure to understand others' beliefs and perspectives as different from one's own are usually quite severe. But again, some especially high-functioning individuals with autism could find work in intellectual or computer-based scientific fields and thrive.

Is there an epidemic of autism? Until the past 15 years or so, the belief was that autism existed maybe 1, 2, or 3 cases out of every 10,000 children; very rare. But in the last 15 years, claims have abounded that autism is skyrocketing in prevalence. In California, for example, the official rates recorded by the state tripled in the early 2000s. But is this a true increase in prevalence, maybe related to vaccinations or other environmental factors? The short answer is this: That's probably not likely. Indeed, in nations that have eliminated all mercury derivatives from vaccines, including the United States, rates of autism have continued to rise well after the changed policies related to the vaccine composition. In the United States, we stopped thimerisol, a mercury derivative, many years ago; but autism has not abated but actually increased in prevalence.

What is happening, certainly, is that a whole spectrum of autism and what we call other "pervasive developmental disorders" are now diagnosed way more than ever before. This could be because of the visibility of the condition, and its clearly established nature in helping to get special education school services. The autism spectrum is better promoted and recognized. High-functioning autism, or Asperger's disorder, is now used to describe youth who might have been given different diagnoses a generation ago: borderline schizophrenia, mild retardation, or other diagnoses.

Here's a provocative alternative idea that could explain a real rise in prevalence called the "Silicon Valley Syndrome," referring, of course, to the microcomputer capital of the United States, in the San Francisco Bay area. The idea is that 2 parents, each of whom may have some autistic tendencies—they might be "computer nerds" with well-developed mathematical and spatial skills, but rather poor social abilities—tend to mate and produce offspring with enhanced genetic risk. The fancy psychological term for this is called "assortative mating"; birds of a feather flocking together, cohabitating, and creating children. This theory may have some validity; it could explain some of the increase in prevalence on autistic disorder in at least some subpopulations.

What are the causes of autism? As I noted a bit earlier in today's lecture, heritability is as high in autism as it is for any psychiatric condition, as high as 90%. Again, there's no "autism gene," but rather a potential host of genes for various forms of this disorder. There could be other biological risk factors in utero that enhance or perpetuate this genetic risk. Contrary to those views that faulty parenting was the cause of autism, consider this: Symptoms of autism are often present from the very earliest months of life. Next, many children with autism actually show secure attachment, the core concept discussed back in Lecture Eight, as long as the coding scheme for attachment in the strange situation takes into account some of the oddities in the child's behavior. Finally, fully 1/4 of children with autism will develop often severe seizures by adolescence or early adulthood. This is a clear signal that something neurological, rather than some purely psychological or family roots, exists for the disorder.

An important sidelight: A subset of children with autism, maybe 20–25%, appear to develop normally during the first 12 months of life, but then tend to regress significantly, losing the speech they had, losing cognitive functions during the second year. It could be that the much larger numbers of vaccinations kids are required to get these days—about twice as many as in the 1970s or '80s—coincide with these symptoms during the second year of life.

For some in this subgroup, their head circumferences, measured with a tape measure, are larger than normal, possibly signifying that one mechanism could be a failure in neuronal pruning, leading to somewhat large and inefficient brains. This is the subject of intensive research.

Simon Baron-Cohen in the United Kingdom has hypothesized that people with autism actually represent an extreme of "male" traits (very logical, very spatial) without compensatory "female" traits (empathy, compassion, and interpersonal concern). This could be one reason, he considers, why autism is at least 4 to 1, male to female, in ratio.

What about treatments? One to one treatments in a therapist's office don't bode well for autism. The most well-documented intervention strategy is intensive, in-home behavioral treatment from a social learning perspective. These include rewards for language skills and social skills; and at least 20 hours per week during the preschool years appear to be necessary to really help autistic kids come out of their shells and make social and language gains. Initial claims that this kind of treatment would essentially cure autism in at least 50% of cases appear to be overstated; that research didn't have randomly assigned control groups. But it is now clear that such early stimulation, early training, and clear rewards can help establish language, cognitive, and behavioral skills that could allow for regular education, not special education, for the rest of the child's school career.

Are medications used for autism? Yes, to help with some of the attentional problems, some of the obsessionality, or tantruming that may accompany autistic disorder. But no medication, as of yet, is anywhere near a primary treatment. A whole range of alternative treatments—ranging from biofeedback to holding therapy to various hormones—have been tried, but with no controlled scientific evidence for effectiveness. It's completely understandable, however, that parents and families would try almost anything for this baffling condition.

What's the overall point? Major difficulties with social connection present huge problems for the development of the mind, autism being a clear example. Finding ways to unlock the isolation and solitariness of individuals with autistic disorder is currently a major clinical and scientific priority nationally. The clear lesson is that if basic social connectedness is lacking, serious mental disorders will be likely to exhibit themselves from the earliest months of life; that's how important social relations and empathy are to our species and our developing minds.

Again, great efforts and large spending are now occurring to find causes of and treatments for autism. It will be essential that these efforts keep in mind the normative pathways to theory of mind, empathy, and social relatedness. We must continue to recognize also that autism occurs on a spectrum; there are many degrees of severity and liability. Thanks for your involvement in this difficult yet fascinating series of lectures on mental disorder.

One other comment: I note a movement that's been proliferating in some quarters called "neurodiversity." The core idea is that atypical or neurodivergent development is a normal human difference; we should recognize it and respect it as any other human variation. Many talented individuals, in this view—albeit maybe nontraditional, somewhat noncommunicative—have autistic features, but we shouldn't give them a label of mental illness. The same reasoning applies, by analogy, to creative people who might be branded as having bipolar disorder, or multi-taskers with ADHD. This is provocative; maybe even a potentially liberating perspective. It places in sharp relief the dimensional continuum way of viewing behavioral deviance as on the same spectrum of normal functioning versus a sharply categorical, discontinuous perspective.

On the other hand, at their extremes, all of the conditions we have been discussing—schizophrenia, mood disorders, ADHD, and autism—are, in my view, clear disorders, deserving of respect but also treatment, given the serious impairments linked to them. It remains to be seen just how tolerant, indeed, we as a species will be with respect to individuals with such behavioral and emotional differences, especially given their continuing presence, at quite high prevalence rates, around the world.

Lecture Twenty-One
Evolution and the Paradox of Mental Illness

Scope:

The major forms of mental disorder are distressingly prevalent, universal across cultures, and highly impairing. Because they carry moderate to high heritability, a paradox is apparent: Wouldn't the risk for mental disorders have been eliminated from the gene pool long ago? This lecture probes important aspects of genetic and evolutionary theory to resolve this paradox.

Outline

I. What we have learned about mental illness appears to convey a large mystery or paradox.

A. Mental disorders are distressingly prevalent, existing as long as human history has been recorded, with its major forms found in every culture on Earth. Overall, moderate to severe mental disorders affect at least a quarter of the world's population.

B. Mental illnesses are highly impairing. Their core symptoms eat away at the most productive years of life, erode healthy identities, affect school and work performance, devastate families, cost the world economy untold billions of dollars each year, and lead to huge personal suffering.

C. The major forms of mental disorder are moderately to strongly heritable. Major depression has a heritability of 30% in males and 40% in females; the heritability of schizophrenia approaches 60%; ADHD, 70–80%; bipolar disorder, 80%; and autism, nearly 90%.

D. It is important to note that the genetic predisposition to mental disturbance exists on a continuum.

E. How can mental illnesses be this prevalent, this impairing, and this heritable—and still have persisted across generations? Shouldn't they have bred themselves out of existence? A close look at key principles of genetic theory and evolutionary theory can help to resolve this apparent paradox.

II. The first answer lies in the concept of heterozygote superiority.

    A. Certain genes come in 2 forms, one dominant allele, capital D, and one recessive allele, small d. The dominant allele, when present, produces the phenotype; the recessive "carries" the phenotype only when there are 2 copies of it.

    B. Because we all carry 2 alleles of each gene, 1 inherited from the mother and 1 from the father, an individual can be a dominant homozygote (DD), a recessive homozygote (dd), or a heterozygote (Dd).

    C. In some cases, the recessive allele of the gene conveys risk for disorder, but heterozygotes have a particular advantage.

    D. Thus, carriers or heterozygotes have a selective reproductive advantage, which outweighs, at a population level, the disadvantage that pertains to rare homozygotes. The recessive allele persists in the population because of heterozygote superiority.

    E. What is the pertinence to mental illness? Even though no mental disorders are dominant or recessive, the same principle doubtless applies: Those with partial risk may have particular advantage.

III. The second answer has to do with the effects of genes. Genes exert complex effects, through gene-gene interactions or gene-environment interactions. A single gene may or not be a risk gene, depending on the surrounding genotype or surrounding environment.

IV. The third answer is that the genes from our genetic heritage, which may have been quite adaptive during earlier parts of human evolutionary history, are no longer adaptive given the current environments in we find ourselves.

V. Overall, evolution and natural selection provide fresh and important perspectives on reasons for the apparent paradox of the continued presence of heritable, highly impairing mental illnesses. The paradox posed at the beginning of this lecture may actually not be so paradoxical.

Suggested Reading:

No book-length account of this topic yet exists, but for some examples see Andreasen, *Brave New Brain*, and Hinshaw, *The Mark of Shame*.

Questions to Consider:

1. What are some of the traits or behavior patterns that may have been adaptive in earlier stages of our species' history but are now considered maladaptive or even signs of mental disorder?

2. Why is the concept of heterozygote superiority significant for understanding the surprising persistence of mental illness throughout human history?

Lecture Twenty-One—Transcript
Evolution and the Paradox of Mental Illness

Today, we address a major paradox: From our last several lectures we know that the major forms of mental disorder are first, quite prevalent; and second, substantially impairing. Third, we've also emphasized that they have anywhere from moderate to strong heritability. But if we put these facts together, we quickly find ourselves embroiled in a paradox, even a major mystery: How could it be the case that mental disorders are passed along through the generations via genes—or, to be precise, as we have learned throughout this course, that the vulnerability to such conditions is transmitted genetically—and be as disabling and impairing as they are, and still persist at the rates they do? In other words, wouldn't these conditions, and the genes that underlie them, simply have bred themselves out of existence? Genes, through natural selection, would have rather quickly disappeared from the gene pool if the mental and emotional conditions for which they provide vulnerability are as impairing as I have presented, right?

The goal of today's lecture is to address this baffling problem. In so doing, we will address some of the complexities of the genetic and evolutionary bases of the human mind. I believe that you'll come away with a deeper appreciation of the origins of the mind, of evolution, and of how genes operate.

Let's first completely understand the paradox: First, adult forms of serious mental illness are distressingly prevalent. Major depression afflicts up 15–20% of women and up to 8–10% of men during their lifetimes. Bipolar disorder, or manic-depressive illness, affects 2% or more of the world's population. If we consider a larger spectrum—of individuals with mood instability, or with what is sometimes called "cyclothymia," a less severe variation of bipolar disorder—that prevalence probably doubles. Schizophrenia is rarer, around 1% of the world's population; but again, if we consider an entire spectrum—for example, of people with paranoia, or markedly disturbed thinking—but without all of the full features of schizophrenia, the number multiplies above 1%. We haven't even addressed anxiety disorders beyond PTSD, which can involve disabling fears; but well beyond specific phobias—like the fear of heights or the fear of snakes—such conditions affect at least 5% and perhaps closer to 10% of the adult population.

Here's an alarming statistic: If we subtract out the comoribidities—that is, the people who have 2 or more conditions; including them would be a kind of double-counting—it appears that 1/4 of the world's population is affected with moderate to severe forms of mental illness in any given one-year period. When we add in milder conditions, like some specific phobias, the number grows to over a third; more than that if we include what's called "lifetime risk" across the entire lifespan. If we restrict ourselves to those most serious conditions involving psychosis, suicidal acts, or highly impairing substance abuse, the number is still more than 1 in 20, about 5 to 6%. First, it's clear that mental illness is not at all rare.

The second point: These conditions have existed in every culture on Earth, and they have been present throughout history as long as we've recorded it. Indeed, for excellent clinical descriptions of most mental disorders, consider the Bible, as well as other historical writings from other different cultures. There are some culturally specific forms of mental disorder—as just one example, running amok, a Filipino/Malaysian syndrome whereby young men go wild with homicidal frenzy—but the serious forms of mental disturbance we've discussed in this course are universal; they're a part of the human condition, again, throughout history and in every culture.

Third, there's strong evidence that mental disturbance is indeed part of our evolutionary heritage, given the moderate to strong heritabilities for all the forms we've discussed. Just to recall: Heritability is that percentage, ranging from 0–100%, signifying how much of the differences or variance across people in a given trait or condition can be explained by genes, rather than environments. Let's review the figures: Major depression has a heritability of about 30% in men and 40% in women. The heritability of schizophrenia approaches 60%. Bipolar disorder has an extremely high heritability of over 80%.

Our fourth point; crucially, in terms of today's lecture: Mental illnesses are quite impairing. Their core symptoms eat away at the most productive years of life, often afflicting individuals during adolescence or early adulthood and then persisting. They can erode healthy identities. They seriously affect school and work performance. They cost the global economy untold hundreds of billions of dollars per year. They can lead to devastation of families and social relationships; they can lead to untold personal suffering. As we discussed earlier, the

Global Burden of Disease reports have shown that among the world's top 10 most devastating illness, mental disorders comprise 5 of these; major depression is now the number 1 most impairing illness on our planet.

Even more specificity is helpful here: Depression produces risk for not only psychological problems, but physical disorders like diabetes and heart disease. Researchers are actively probing the relevant mechanisms, but it's clear that depression leads to cascades of hormonal and even immunological problems. Bipolar disorder, as we emphasized, is lethal in terms of its ultra-high risk of promoting suicide; again, if untreated, half of individuals with this disorder will make a series attempt, and 20% will actually complete suicide. Schizophrenia erodes rational thinking, emotional control, and motivation; loss of economic productivity, loss of identity, and loss of relationships all add up to heartbreak and more for family members.

I have focused for now on the adult disorders in the arguments I've just made; but the same applies to the child conditions we've discussed, ADHD and autism. ADHD, to quickly review, has a prevalence of 6–8%; it's present in all cultures that have compulsory education; it's 70–80% heritable; and it's quite devastating with regard to academics, peer relationships, and the risk of accidental injury. Autism, while much rarer, is now recognized around the world and afflicts almost 1% of all children in some form. It's extremely heritable, up to 90%, and it creates serious disabilities in social relatedness and independence.

With all of these facts in mind, we're just about ready to try to solve this paradox. But I'd like to first briefly revisit the neurodiversity concept noted at the end of our last lecture. Here's the point: Realizing the utter impairment that can accrue from mental disorder, it gets really difficult—for me at least, and I know others—to consider that major depression, bipolar illness, and schizophrenia, as well as ADHD and autism, are simply instances of diversity or neurodiversity. Can we really believe that they're just a little further out on the bell curve than normal variations, keeping in mind those serious life impairments I just reviewed? Sometimes the neurodiversity perspective can downplay or ignore the devastation that these conditions really incur in their full form.

But there is, in fact, real evidence behind the belief that the major forms of mental illnesses are spectrum conditions, they range in severity from mild to severe; all the evidence is now pointing in that direction. Here are 2 key points: Number one, we will continue to be challenged as a society—with regard to the statistical model first introduced in Lecture Sixteen—to find the right cutoff point, the right diagnostic threshold, for considering what is mentally disordered and what falls on the other side. The stakes are high; we don't want to over-label and find mental disorder everywhere; we want to avoid false positive decisions. But on the other hand, missing true cases could lead to personal and family tragedy if we don't identify and get treatment; false negatives could constitute a problem that's even worse.

Another point: The spectrum idea is really intriguing when we consider the genetic liabilities for mental illness; in fact, the genetic liabilities may themselves be on a continuum. As we've discussed, there's no particular gene for any specific form of mental disorder. Genetic vulnerability appears quantitative itself: Those individuals with a perhaps a few more risk alleles that confer liability—especially if the environmental context is threatening—may succumb, but those with a couple fewer risk alleles may not, particularly if the environment is supportive. Genes, therefore, yield a quantitative, continuous risk for mental disorders; not a yes/no, one gene/one disorder absolute certainty. This gives us a hint about why mental disorders might have persisted through the ages, despite their clear impairments; in other words, the genes underlying them may not be problematic, and actually could be advantageous from the point of natural selection if they are present in relatively low quantities. Let's go on; I'll try to make this as clear as possible.

Let's recap the puzzle: How can mental disorders continue to exist at such high rates when the underlying vulnerability genes should be likely to have been selected out of the population, given the strong impairments that they typically produce? If natural selection really works, wouldn't these conditions just have bred themselves out of existence? Look at how impairing these conditions are, once again; it's unlikely, for example, that too many people with schizophrenia or autism, or the severest forms of depression, would be likely to reproduce as much as those without such conditions.

Can a close look at genes and evolution help to resolve this mystery and paradox? I believe so; here are the 3 core ideas we'll focus on today: Number one, there's a concept with a daunting name called "heterozygote superiority." What's a "heterozygote," first, before we figure out what's superior? Heterozygotes are individuals who have— remember from high-school biology—combinations of alleles; so we might inherit from our male parent one form and from our female parent the other form. In classic cases, there could be a dominant ("D") gene, and the other form is recessive ("d"). When the dominant allele is present, it produces the dominant phenotype, even if the other allele is recessive. The recessive allele "carries" the day with a phenotype only when there are 2 copies of it. An individual could be a dominant homozygote ("DD"), a recessive homozygote ("dd"), or a heterozygote (the combination of "Dd").

As an example, brown eye color is determined by a dominant gene and blue eye color by a recessive gene. "BB" and "Bb" individuals will therefore in the classic case have brown eyes; only "bb" will have blue eyes. If both parents are themselves heterozygotes, 25% of their offspring will be homozygotes for the recessive form. For many traits, like eye color, blends do exist—hazel eyes; or green eyes like my own—but let's stick to the classic case for the moment.

Here's the crucial point: In some instances, the recessive allele conveys serious risk for disorder. Here's a good example: a disease called "sickle cell anemia." This is a blood disorder with particularly high prevalence among African and African-American populations. How do you get sickle cell anemia? Only one way: You inherit the recessive allele from both parents; so you have "ss." In these cases, the resulting disease—which we call "sickle cell anemia"—is potentially lethal; the red blood cells are not round and healthy, but instead weak, with a kind of sickle, crescent shape. What's the heritability of sickle cell anemia? It's 100%; it's a single-gene, recessive condition—all of the variability in whether or not you get it is related to genes—and it's often fatal at even young ages. Children or young adults are at risk for many serious medical complications related to their cardiovascular functioning.

Sickle cell anemia, by any rational perspective, should have bred itself out of existence long ago. But here's the real story: Heterozygotes— those who have the "Ss" genotype—have actually a particular advantage. In tropical climates—for example in Africa, where mosquito-borne malaria is a potentially lethal infectious disease— these heterozygotes who don't get sickle-cell anemia but whose red blood cells are slightly different from the "SS" homozygotes have an immunity to malaria; in other words, the slightly different red blood cell phenotype of the heterozygotes renders it resistant to malaria, a huge selective advantage. In all, "carriers" or heterozygotes have a reproductive advantage, and this outweighs numerically, at the population level, the disadvantage that pertains to rarer homozygotes. There are many more carriers (heterozygotes), and their immunity to malaria preserves more genes than the rarer, homozygotic cases of sickle cell anemia. The recessive allele persists in the population, even though when it exists in the homozygotic form ("ss") it can be devastating. This is really a revelation.

The immediate question is: Does this pertain at all to mental illness? Remember, no mental illnesses are single-gene dominant or recessive conditions; as we've discussed, they're polygenic, resulting from multiple alleles of multiple genes. But the same principle doubtless applies: Those with partial risk may have a particular advantage; those with some genetic liability may prosper. Is there evidence? Think of bipolar disorder: For example, here, biological relatives of people with bipolar illness are highly likely to be successful socioeconomically, with business, academic, and creative talents. This has been shown in several large representative studies. Reproductive advantage could accrue from partial genetic risk for this otherwise devastating condition; and remember, the heritability of bipolar illness is quite high, 80%. It could also be the case that "carriers," or those with a partial loading for schizophrenia, have particular ways of construing the world that are slightly askew, perhaps even innovative.

What about depression? Mild forms of this condition, maybe reflecting a partial genetic loading, could yield particular sensitivity, reflectiveness, or ability to bond with others deeply, whereas others without such loading do not have these same traits. Partial loading could, again, conceivably be adaptive in an evolutionary sense. We showed back in Lecture Nineteen that there was selective advantage for some of our ancestors with risk alleles for ADHD; remember the 7-repeat allele of the Dopamine, type 4 receptor. Such risk-takers may well have had an advantage in changing climates and migrating to new lands.

Overall, those with some amount of genetic risk for mental disorder may actually have a selective advantage, outweighing, at the overall level of natural selection, the clear disadvantages and impairments for those with the full loading. This concept of heterozygote superiority is our first candidate for helping to understand why mental disorders have survived in human history as long as they have. Some of the paradox of the high rates of mental illness throughout the history of our species may not be quite so paradoxical after all.

What's the second potential answer to this paradox in history? It has to do with the following: Single genes may have a different action from that same gene in combination or in concert with other genes or in different environments. Not only might there be 2 or more alleles of the same gene, but, as we've emphasized throughout the course, it may take multiple genes working together to create the risk for mental disorder. Think of this: A single gene acting in relative isolation could provide a beneficial phenotype in a certain environment; but that same gene, when it now acts in combination with certain forms of other genes, may have a deleterious effect. Certain genes produce risks for mental disorders only in the presence of certain environments or certain contexts; this is the phenomenon known as "gene-environment interaction," further complicating the picture.

I'm getting abstract, so let's look at some core examples: Let's go back to the Dopamine, Type 4 receptor gene (the DRD4 gene). It codes for the fourth type of the dopamine postsynaptic receptor in the brain; remember, receptors are proteins and genes code for the construction of proteins. This gene is polymorphic; it exists in several different allelic forms. One, the 7-repeat allele, produces, on average, tendency toward sensation seeking and risk taking. Individuals high on these traits may have, again, migrated or "pushed the frontier" when the Ice Age receded; this allele, in fact, increased in frequency for those humans who migrated across the Bering Strait land mass from Asia to North America. In this sense, acting "on its own," this allele may well have been advantageous, at least in certain environments. But in the presence of other "risk" alleles from other genes—other genes coding for dopamine, norepinephrine, or serotonin—this 7-repeat allele of DRD4 actually predicts the development of ADHD in modern society. Genes acting alone versus genes compounded by other genes: The latter could magnify or change the effect of the 7-repeat allele, yielding high risk for ADHD.

A protective, helpful, or potentially adaptive gene, in relative isolation, may not be protective at all when other genetic variants interact with it. We call this "gene-by-gene interaction"; in the lingo, these are "epistatic effects." Let's not forget gene-by-environment interactions, back from Lecture Fifteen. The basic principle is this: with the example, certain alleles of serotonin genes, certain alleles of COMT genes, or genes for other neuroactive substances convey increased risk for mental illness only in the presence of certain adverse life circumstances. The short-arm form of the serotonin transporter gene increases risk for depression only when the individual was either maltreated in childhood or had a large number of negative loss events in adolescence or early adulthood.

What's the overall point? Genes exert complex effects through gene-gene interactions or gene-environment interactions. A single gene may or not be a "risk" gene, depending on the surrounding genotype or the surrounding environment. That gene could, in fact, convey risk in certain environments, but be quite adaptive in others; some genes are actually plasticity genes.

Again, because that gene may be helpful when acting alone, or in certain life circumstances, it may well have staying power through the evolutionary history of our species. When we view things in this way, it's again not so much of a mystery, after all, as to why certain genes conferring risk for mental illness may have persisted throughout our species.

Here's a third principle and a third mechanism. The point is this: Certain genes from our genetic heritage, which may have been quite adaptive during earlier parts of human evolutionary history, aren't adaptive in our current environments. They might actually be quite maladaptive in the current contexts in which we find ourselves—and, in fact, that we've created for ourselves—in the very recent past of our species. Back to "Darwin's moths": Remember, white moths in England were the "healthy" ones; their genetically-controlled color protected them from predators on their homes on white lichens on British trees. But as the Industrial Revolution led to pollution, as tree bark darkened, there was now a selective advantage for those initially rare mutants with black coloring. What was an adaptive genetic trait drastically changed once the environment changed; and what was maladaptive in mutant form became adaptive. We've found a reversal in recent years: With pollution controls in England, the situation has again reversed; moths with the gene contributing to white color have again flourished.

What does this have to do with the human mind and human mental disorder? Let's consider a mild form of mental disorder, snake phobia: It was undoubtedly adaptive in early human history to have been quickly frightened by reptiles, snakes, and other such life forms. These kinds of stimuli automatically elicit fear emotions, motivating the urge to flee. Primates or humans who have never encountered snakes are automatically fearful of them; it's almost built into our genes. Better to be safe than sorry, from the perspective of the behavioral program encoded in our genes to abandon ship when such a creature is sighted; one missed detection could have produced fatality. But today, with our urbanized environment, we call such fears "phobias" and we treat them with behavior therapy or medications. In other words, what was adaptive previously in human history is now not at all adaptive because our environments have changed so radically; houses, urbanization, cities, and the like.

Here's an example from medicine: The ability to metabolize and utilize high-fat meals was clearly advantageous during those periods of human history when food was scarce and energy was needed for sudden hunts, attacks, or retreats. But today's world is much more sedentary, and the "taste" sort of in our genes for certain high-cholesterol, high-fat, or high-sugar foods may now be life-threatening, as they can lead to atherosclerosis, coronaries, and diabetes. From this perspective, there are no inherently "good" genes or adaptive genes, or no inherently "bad" or maladaptive genes; rather, genes convey selective advantage or disadvantage depending on the shifting environments or contexts in which a species lives. What was clearly adaptive during earlier times of our evolutionary history may not at all be adaptive or advantageous today.

Here's a counterexample: In some cases of schizophrenia, copying errors of genes during meiosis may lead to deletions of major chunks of genes, and schizophrenia-like symptoms can emerge. These are really harmful; in all likelihood, these don't survive in any Darwinian sense through natural selection. But, just about all of our genes and their various alleles would not have been promoted and preserved in our gene pool unless they carried some selective advantage, at least back in the "environments of evolutionary adaptation," as they are called, from 100,000 years ago.

If you think of this perspective, this is like the ecological model back in Lecture Sixteen. Mental disorder is not entirely biological and genetic, nor entirely environmental; it results from a mismatch—in this case, between certain genotypes, naturally selected throughout our species' history—and our current environment.

What's the overall answer to today's mystery? The paradox may have somewhat disappeared. Mental disorders, particularly those with substantial heritability, may survive in the gene pool because first, of a form of heterozygote superiority: Genes that convey partial risk may be quite adaptive, but the genotype leading to the full condition could actually be harmful. The lesser-frequency allele thrives because of the advantage of this partial genetic loading. And, genes acting in relative isolation could yield quite different effects from those that are modified by other genes; and certain alleles may cause little or no harm in one environment—even an advantage—where they might be quite devastating in other settings, as we know from the phenomenon of gene-gene interaction. Finally, genes promoting behaviors that served an adaptive function earlier in human history may not be so advantageous in our current, highly urbanized, and in many ways artificial settings and contexts within which most of us live.

Knowledge about genes and evolution can therefore shed light on a great puzzle and help us to understand that mental disorders are not the terrible, inherently flawed, subhuman aberrations that they are too often stereotyped and portrayed as being; but rather are part of our genetic, evolutionary, and ecological heritage. A lot of the mystery and terror related to mental illness may recede when we bring evolution to bear on the problem. I do hope that these concepts have proven illuminating. What seemed like the ultimate paradox maybe isn't now so paradoxical after all when we think of genes, evolution, and the human mind. The perspective today shows the linkages more clearly than ever between the mind's strengths and its potential weaknesses.

If evolution helps us to understand how psychological weaknesses are intertwined with psychological strengths, what about social strengths and weaknesses? In our next lecture, we look at the evolutionary origins of the human mind in social terms: the evolutionary origins of human culture.

Lecture Twenty-Two
Roots of Religion, Aggression, and Prejudice

Scope:

This lecture features evolutionary perspectives on 3 key issues related to the human mind: the overwhelming tendency for humans to have religious beliefs, the levels of human aggression that exist, and the strong proclivity to stigmatize fellow humans with physical and behavioral differences. We discuss the core human tendency to show prejudice, discrimination, and stigma toward those with different skin colors, national origins, or behavioral patterns than our own. Exclusion modules in our minds may have developed in order to prevent runaway social bonds.

Outline

I. Humans have an overwhelming tendency to believe in supernatural powers, to posit a creator, and to hold religious beliefs.

    A. All known societies have been permeated with religion. Even in modern America, over 90% of the general public professes belief in higher powers.

    B. From an evolutionary perspective, capacities related to religious beliefs include symbolic communication; language and narrative; a sense of continuity between past, present, and future; the tendency to attribute causes and intentionality to events in the world; the ability to ascribe mental states to others; and perhaps the ability to experience emotions like awe.

    C. Can we consider religious beliefs and practices as a true adaptation? Or are they a by-product related to theory of mind, agency attributions, or symbolic skills emerging in early humans?

    D. In the early 21st century, controversy accompanied the hypothesis that there is a specific "God gene"— that is, a specific mutation, which spread, creating belief in higher powers. It is unlikely that any 1 gene underlies such complex beliefs.

E. Other views include the perspective that religion emerged from primates' intense attachment bonds with early caregivers, fueling empathy and a deep need for belongingness; and the assertion that, over time, humans have created deistic entities less vengeful and more compassionateas the result of social structures favoring cooperation.

II. A fundamental debate centers humans social behavior; are humans fundamentally good, helpful, and prosocial, but swayed by modeling, learning, and even the media to be selfish and aggressive?

    A. Social learning views emphasize the learned nature of aggression; psychodynamic perspectives feature their instinctual basis.

    B. There are pervasive human tendencies to expand into new territories, impose the victorious group's will on and enslave those groups who are vanquished, and disrupt the natural environment severely. But we also negotiate to meet our needs, rather than throw our weight around.

    C. Developmentally, the most aggressive members of our species, in terms of the sheer number of aggressive acts, are 1–2 year olds! It is not that some children start to display aggression during the preschool years, but rather a small percentage of youth, about 5% of boys and 1% of girls, fail to develop brakes on aggression.

    D. Whatever the ultimate roots of human aggression, if our species is to continue to evolve, some better ways of curbing aggression must be enacted.

III. What are the roots of human diversity?

    A. Humans living closer to the equator were advantaged if they carried genes that protected them from the Sun's intense ultraviolet rays—that is, if they were able to produce enough melanin to have a darker skin color. When humans migrated to northern latitudes, mutations allowing more vitamin D to enter the body supported lighter skin color.

    B. Personality traits in humans emerged from similar traits in other mammals; we have been selected for variability in such traits.

IV. Despite advantages that accrue from diversity and despite the deeply ingrained tendencies for humans to be social and gregarious, there are naturally selected limitations on indiscriminate sociability.

   A. If humans are indiscriminately social, they may become infected or infested—or exploited, falling victim to those from hostile "outgroups." There is therefore strong likelihood of a core tendency for humans to reject, withdraw from, punish, and stigmatize those whose behaviors signal "outgroup" status.

   B. Stigma is a term from ancient Greece signifying a literal brand or mark placed on traitors or slaves. Today's meaning is more psychological, incorporating stereotypes, prejudice, discrimination, and a global branding of all negative attributes of an individual to group status.

   C. The most stigmatized attributes in current society are homelessness, substance abuse, and mental illness.

   D. It would appear that simply attributing mental illness to a medical or genetic model would greatly reduce stigma. However, evidence exists that such attributions may actually fuel punitive responses.

   E. Communicating the interactive influences on behavioral diversity—and framing diversity in terms of narratives and life stories—may be an antidote to such tendencies to dehumanize and stigmatize.

Suggested Reading:

King, *Evolving God.*

Lorenz, *On Aggression.*

Thornicroft, *Shunned.*

Wright, *The Evolution of God.*

Questions to Consider:

1. What are the evolutionary bases of both religious beliefs and aggressive behaviors—and what are the cultural, learned components of each?

2. Why would attributing mental illness to deviant genes lead, paradoxically, to harsh rather than empathic responses from fellow humans?

Lecture Twenty-Two—Transcript
Roots of Religion, Aggression, and Prejudice

Our last lecture focused on intriguing lessons from evolution and natural selection about the persistence of mental disorder across human history. Today, we examine how evolution can help us understand wider aspects of human culture, with emphasis on 3 core issues: First, throughout history and across all cultures, why have humans been so prone to believe in higher powers and to be religious? Second, how aggressive are we as a species? Third, in what ways has natural selection placed brakes on our intensely social nature, and can that tendency help us to understand prejudice and stigma against fellow humans? These are some big and important questions, so we'd better get started.

Let's begin with a huge, important, and provocative topic: that of the human tendency to believe in supernatural powers, to posit a creator, and to be religious. Of course, this topic could easily take up not only today's entire lecture but our entire course. Religion has many aspects; but for this discussion, a basic definition of religious beliefs and behaviors is that they are related to supernatural powers with "agency" to affect human behaviors. It's clear that these beliefs and practices have appeared in at least some form since we became a species, based primarily on evidence from burial rituals existing from 125,000 or so years ago. Much more elaborate organization of religious practices emerged with the advent of agriculture and civilization around 10,000–12,000 years ago. All known societies have been permeated with religion. Even in apparently secular modern America, over 90% of the general public professes belief in higher powers.

The comments to follow are not predicated on the controversial topic of whether there is or is not a higher being, and if so of what sort, and what your beliefs may or may not be. Rather, let's consider this nearly universal human tendency to have such beliefs and associated religious practices. Number one: From the perspective of evolution, what capacities would be needed to hold such religious beliefs? One would be symbolic communication, including language and narrative. A second would be the ability to have a sense of continuity between past, present, and future. A third is the tendency to attribute causes and intentionality to events in the world; and more specifically, to sense a mysterious, powerful force operating behind everyday events.

©2010 The Teaching Company.

Number 4 would be the ability to ascribe mental states to others, even inanimate objects. Perhaps 5 is the ability to experience complex emotions like a sense of awe.

We know that primates have abilities in some of these areas; indeed, chimps have incredible cognitive abilities and capacities. They and other primates have elements of empathy and even theory of mind. But the question here, as in other areas of the mind, is how continuous or discontinuous the jump is with the advent of modern *Homo sapiens*. Language, symbolization, and abstraction, and our huge tendency to attribute minds and intentions to others—even to inanimate objects— are major contenders for uniquely human skills, which may have helped to propel religious beliefs, practices, and behaviors.

Let's focus more specifically on "agency detection" and causal attribution: All human children begin to do this as early as one-and-a-half years of age. In other words, we are a species that sees personal meaning, control, and agency (a sense of action) in lots of natural events, and we instinctively do so from very young ages. When faced with the wonders of nature, or the terror of death, it may have been natural for such a species to begin to attribute human-like qualities to objects in the world and to acts of nature.

Consider this, another huge point: Human commitment to group living may have played a key role. As social group size increased from roughly 50 in chimps to the more common mean number of 150 in humans—a point we discussed earlier in this course—there was great need for means of exerting social control. Religious powers could serve as a true "higher power" to enforce restraints on selfishness, identification with an ingroup, to promote strong social bonds, and to incur a moral imperative to follow rules. With the more recent advent of agriculture and permanent settlements in the past 10,000–12,000 years, hierarchical societies emerged based on division of labor. More elaborated religions served, in part, the objectives of maintaining social order and sometimes justifying hugely powerful royalty. We can't forget humans' narrative abilities, the mythic skills described by Merlin Donald, which not only convey meaning through story-telling, but also, given humans' abilities to project backwards and forwards in time, confront us directly with suffering and the prospect of our own deaths

With these capacities and abilities in mind, what are some of the forms of early religious beliefs; we're in the land of speculation here, as no fossil record directly appears? Matt Rossano of Southeastern Louisiana University posits that even before modern humans emerged around 150,000 years ago, ecstatic rituals may have promoted social bonding among hominids, altering consciousness at the same time. As we described before, burial practices appear to be a sign of beliefs in an afterlife, some early religious beliefs; clear evidence is found from at least 125,000 years ago. No other primates show signs of this practice. Shamanistic practices of healing through getting in touch with the spirit world seem to be another indicator; some evidence of these practices in the past 100,000 years exists.

Can we consider religious beliefs and practices to be a true adaptation, which have been naturally selected? Some evolutionary psychologists believe so, given that religion appears to have played such a key role in social bonding among hunter-gatherers and other early humans. But others consider religion a byproduct, what is sometimes called an "exaptation," a function that is linked with a true adaptation, but it's not naturally selected itself. Steven Pinker, for example, considers religious beliefs just such an exaptation, perhaps a byproduct of our abilities to have a theory of mind—imputing intentions and beliefs to others, even to inanimate objects—kind of gone wild.

Fourth, we noted earlier that the proneness to be religious is at least moderately heritable, so there's some genetic tendency underlying individual differences in religious convictions and in belief of some kind of higher power. But the particular form of religious beliefs one has are virtually zero in terms of heritability; these differences are clearly the result of socialization and family practice.

In the early 21st century, there was a splash of controversy accompanying the hypothesis that there might be a specific "God gene"; a specific gene related to neurotransmission, which was proposed to predict the tendency toward mystical feelings leading to religious, spiritual beliefs. Recent science has provided a lot of skepticism about such a single-gene idea; but the tendency to have such beliefs does appear partly heritable, perhaps related to multiple genes linked to imagination, attribution of intent to natural forces, and other mental capacities.

Thinking of microevolution back from Lecture Seven, could it be that certain genes promoting high brain efficiency in modern humans were, in fact, linked to precursors to religious tendencies, a belief in an afterlife, or more advanced burial rituals? This is a provocative question, indeed.

Finally, interest in the evolutionary origins of religion is, if anything, intensifying these days. In 2007, Barbara King's book, *Creating God*, argues that religion emerged from primates' intense attachment bonds with early caregivers, fueling empathy and a deep need for belongingness. In 2009, Robert Wright wrote *The Evolution of God*, and he argued that, despite the clear evidence for evolutionary origins of religious tendencies, over the period of recorded history, humans have created deistic entities less and less vengeful and more and more tolerant and compassionate as the direct result of social structures that tended to favor cooperation.

Next topic: What about human social behavior, including aggression; another huge topic that could form the basis for an entire course? Are humans fundamentally good, helpful, and prosocial, but swayed by modeling, learning, and even the media to be selfish and aggressive? This is a view in keeping with many social learning perspectives going all the way back to Lecture Five. Or, on the other hand, are we born with selfish, primal instincts, at odds with the larger social group, requiring huge amounts of socialization to curb these aggressive tendencies? This is a distinctly Freudian, psychodynamic perspective, also introduced back in Lecture Five.

There's no way to address all the evidence, and controversy reigns in this area. In *Guns, Germs, and Steel*, Jared Diamond chronicles the human tendencies, over and over again in recorded history, to expand into new territories, impose the victorious group's will on and even enslave those groups who are vanquished, and all too often, to disrupt the natural environment severely. Are we really destined to be territorial and exploitative? On the other hand, among many others, social psychologist Roy Baumeister notes in *The Cultural Animal* that what's amazing really is that most humans are not aggressive most of the time. We negotiate to meet our needs, rather than throw our weight around. My colleague Dacher Keltner of UC Berkeley, in his book *Born to be Good*, emphasizes the ways in which natural selection has actually prepared us to cooperate, to fall in love, co-parent, and much more.

Here's a helpful perspective, I believe; it's really developmental: Who are the most aggressive members of our species, in terms of the sheer number of aggressive acts they commit? These are 1- to 2-year-olds. It's normative as the self develops and a sense of "agency" at this age, kids call out "mine" and grab objects and display rampant territoriality. The conceptual and clinical question is not why some children start to display aggression during the preschool years, it's instead why a small percentage of youth—about 5% of boys, about 1% of girls— fail to develop brakes on aggression. These are what are called "early starters," who are really early "persisters" from the toddler years, and are vastly likely to become delinquent. Such youngsters typically have difficult temperaments; insecure or disorganized attachments; early problems with executive functions; and they're parented by caregivers with high levels of stress, perhaps mental disorders, or substance abuse, who are either extremely authoritarian, extremely permissive, or both in combination. There are multiple, interacting risk factors related to why this small percentage of youth don't show the normative pattern of refraining from aggression year by year after toddlerhood.

Whatever the ultimate roots of human aggression, one thing, I believe, is quite clear: If our species is to continue to evolve, some better ways of putting brakes on aggression must be enacted, given, of course, the huge technological advances that make modern weaponry likely to annihilate a major portion of humans if not our entire population. This could well be our most fundamental problem to solve as a species.

After religion and aggression—2 icebreaker topics at cocktail parties, I might add—our third topic more specifically deals with how evolutionary theory and evolutionary psychology could help us to understand one kind of aggression and exclusion in humans, this is the form based on prejudice towards those who aren't members of our primary ingroups.

Let's start: We humans constitute a species. We mate with one another and we produce viable offspring, despite our differences in color, size, other physical features, and differences in our behavior. This is one of the most common definitions, of course, of a species: Members of a biological group who can viably reproduce.

Back in Lecture Seven, we noted some of the evolutionary roots of human physical diversity. As just one example, skin color: Our predecessors, who lived relatively close to the equator in Africa, evolved less and less fur or body hair. But within the past 12,000 years or so, those humans who migrated to live in far Northern Europe experienced mutations in several genes related to skin color. These produced lighter-colored skin, which allows greater absorption of ultraviolet rays from the sun, helpful in producing Vitamin D. In regions where sunlight was limited, this was actually a selective advantage. Other mutations led to genotypes promoting diverse types of behavior: People differ in the degrees or amounts of the Big Five personality traits of openness, conscientiousness, extraversion and sociability, agreeableness versus aggression, and neuroticism. Remember, each of these has a heritability of approximately 50%.

As a sidelight: Comparative personality research reveals that dogs, as well as many other species, show individual differences in behavioral traits that look a lot like many of the Big Five personality traits. As many of you dog owners undoubtedly know, some dogs and dog breeds are neurotic, some are quite extraverted; they can also differ quite a bit on agreeableness versus hostility. This underscores the point that evolution tends to preserve key structures and functions across species. Human personality didn't originate anew or afresh, but rather built on preserved personality and temperamental mechanisms from other species from which we evolved.

How does all of this relate to aggression or prosocial behavior? Number 1, if we weren't intensely social as a species, we wouldn't procreate and we wouldn't benefit from culture. Without attachment bonds between parent and child, our minds would not have the protection and nurturance needed for their development of plasticity. We clearly need others—families, bands, tribes, communities—for protection, for food sharing, and in the most recent past of our species' history, agricultural and economic support.

As we have discussed earlier, the view espoused most systematically by Roy Baumeister and Merlin Donald is that culture is not only a byproduct of evolution, but our brains and human culture coevolved. Once culture began to teach innovations, those humans who were optimally influenced by culture would have been those who survived, thrived, and reproduced. This is a kind of "ratchet effect." Think of those wrenches that turn the bolt, but then when you swing them back for reloading, they don't lose any ground; progress escalates. In this view, human evolution is predicated on the ability to benefit from culture. Recall also anthropologist Robin Dunbar, who argued that brain size, language, and social group size all coevolved.

How social and how cultural are we as a species? For one thing, perhaps the most incredible deprivation a human can have is to be cut off completely from others. Those who have been in solitary confinement, as just an example, have stated that this experience is far worse than any physical torture. We're a social species to the max, with deep needs for connection. But—and this is a critical "but"— despite the deeply ingrained tendencies for we humans to be social and gregarious, it was also essential, in terms of natural selection, for humans to have some brakes placed on these tendencies. If we had been completely indiscriminately social, we may have become infected or infested, or cheated or exploited; falling victim to those from ill or hostile "outgroups."

Evolutionary psychologists have posited this: Certain mental modules have evolved in order for humans to be able to navigate a perilous but essential interpersonal journey; to find a middle ground between on the one hand bonding with all others and always seeking close contact, and on the other, being wary of social connections that could put us at risk. The evolutionary psychology hypothesis is that naturally selected cognitive modules were formed, propelling humans to reject, withdraw from, punish, and even exploit or eliminate those whose behaviors signal "outgroup" status, not being a member of one's primary family, community, or nation. Here are the 3 most likely triggers posed by evolutionary psychology for such "exclusion modules": Number one, signs in another human of contagion or contamination. This process clearly has been conserved from other species: Animals that excessively groom are often shunned; this could be a sign of potential contamination. We tend to fear and isolate fellow humans who may infect or infest us; think of leper colonies, the emotion of disgust is often raised.

A second exclusion module is linked to signs of exploitation or "low social capital." If we believe that someone can't offer us much in return for our social investment, or even worse, if they may rip us off or cheat us, we are likely to punish and exclude them. Much discussion, in fact, occurs in evolutionary psychology about highly evolved "cheating detection modules" in humans; how exquisitely attuned we are to being cheated or exploited by others. Think, for example, of media outrage against deadbeat dads or welfare cheaters.

Third, an exclusion model tends to exist against those with what we call a different "tribal" status: different skin color, custom, or religion. Here, we tend to be harshly punitive, and even exploitative of those with such differences; we often try to eliminate them from the gene pool. Think of genocide, even Hitler's Germany: His goals were to rid the Earth not only of Jewish individuals but gays and lesbians, the "mentally defective" (those with mental retardation), and those with serious mental illness. Consider the vast and depressing history of human warfare, religious crusades, ethnic cleansing, and the like. We wish to vanquish, dominate, or even annihilate the oppressed group, lest they oppress us; and we develop a set of cognitive strategies to tell ourselves that we are superior to these outgroups.

Here's an important concept along these lines: It's that of "stigma." This is a term from ancient Greece signifying a literal brand or mark placed on traitors or slaves. Everyone at the agora, the Greek marketplace, would therefore be able to recognize in an instant those members of society who were outcasts, not really deserving of being full members of that society. (The anxiety disorder called "agoraphobia" literally means "fear of the marketplace," intense anxiety about being out in public.) Today's meaning of stigma is more psychological, involving less overt, but still powerful, means of branding, noticing, resisting, and resenting members of disfavored groups.

The first aspect of stigma is stereotypes. These are uniform categorizations of all members of a group; they're very cognitive in nature. For me, at UC Berkeley, we have stereotypes against Stanford, our rival school. Stereotypes may contain a germ of truth but they do deny any individuality to the person in question. A second aspect is prejudice; literally, prejudging others. I may now come to form intense dislike of Stanford professors and students, and even their despised team color (red) versus Berkeley's deep blue and gold. Prejudices amplify stereotypes into the domain of negative emotion. Then third, there's actual discrimination. My group will tend now to limit the rights of the stereotyped and despised "outgroup," or even punishes them. Cal Berkeley students deface the property of Stanford buildings and attempt to "steal the Axe," which goes to the victor of the Big Game. At a much more serious level, we may disallow people of different skin color from voting, renting, or marrying. We may torture those of different religious affiliations, especially if we believe that they convey actual threat. We hope for a public conversion, justifying our own deeply-held beliefs.

But stigma goes beyond all 3 of these aspects. If I stigmatize people in a devalued group, I probably stereotype them, I have prejudice against them, and I'm likely to discriminate against them; but I also tend to view all aspects of their minds and behaviors, their entire being, in terms of their degraded group status. Stigma brands the totality of the person, and I may actually come to see the stigmatized individual as less than fully human. We know from history that dehumanization is a major step toward extremely harsh treatment of or even extermination of those in outgroups. Members of stigmatized groups are quite likely to be aware of their own stigmatized status, and they can be prone to engage in self-stigma, taking on some of this negative valuation internally.

If there are naturally selected modules driving us to stigmatize those we believe are contagious, who are cheaters, or of a different "tribe," are we doomed to exploit or stigmatize outgroup members? But recall, we humans can regulate our emotions; we can show compassion and reciprocal altruism. It may take some concerted effort to transcend these naturally selected exclusion tendencies. Reducing automatic biases is not an easy task; fear and stigma could emerge at a very basic, automatic level. I note that not all human diversity is good or productive; we can and we should ensure that our fellow humans uphold basic human values. But the issue is being able to think clearly about tolerance for diversity, rather than succumb to automatic, quick, implicit, and ingrained biases.

What are the conditions or attributes most likely to be stigmatized in current society? Clear evidence exists that the most stigmatized attributes are, in fact, homelessness, substance abuse, and mental illness, even more than ethnic or racial status. The American public knows much more about mental disorder than it did back in the 1950s, but national surveys reveal that there is actually an increase in the last 50 years in our desire to keep distance from people displaying the symptoms of serious mental illness, or those even with the label of "mentally ill." Why on Earth would that be?

Despite the clear humanitarian reasons for closing just about all of our nation's mental hospitals across the last 50 years, the result in too many cases has been a large number of people with serious mental disturbance on the streets, without adequate treatment, sometimes homeless. In addition, newspapers, TV, and the internet still tend to depict people with mental disorders in very stereotyped fashion, emphasizing violence and incompetence. Many people's worst fears include losing their own mind, becoming afflicted with dyscontrol, or being taken advantage of; mental illness may serve as a painful reminder of our key vulnerabilities.

Along these lines, wouldn't it seem reasonable to assume that if we just attributed mental illness to a medical/genetic model, this would reduce stigma? If we call mental illnesses "brain diseases," blame will just go away; we should adapt a naturalistic perspective, this argument goes. Indeed, from social psychology, what we call "attribution theory"—related to humans' search for causes of or attributions for behavior—tells us this: When behavior is negative and when the observer believes that the individual in question could have controlled it, reactions are harshly negative; but if that negative behavior is beyond personal control, observers may feel compassion and support. So, the argument goes, attributing mental disorder to genetic or other biological factors that are clearly beyond the individual's personal control should reduce stigma. This would make sense, given what we know about the moderate to high heritabilities for mental disorders as we've repeatedly discussed.

But research shows that these kinds of attributions could actually fuel punitive responses. In research conducted in the late 1990s, for example, college students were randomly assigned, before interacting with another student, to one of 2 "scripts" allegedly written by this interaction partner. First was the biogenetic condition: The partner's essay stated that he or she had a mental illness and that doctors had explained that genes and biochemistry were the main causes, and medication was the main treatment. The second condition was the psychosocial condition, where the essay stated that the cause was life stress, family factors, and that psychological therapy was the main treatment. As would be expected, the subjects reported less blame for those in the first biogenetic condition. But subsequently, when they interacted with the partner—who was really a confederate of the experimenter—they delivered more electric shock to the partner in that biogenetic condition when the partner didn't succeed in a learning task.

What gives; why would this paradoxical finding be present? This the exact opposite of what attribution theory would predict. Here are a couple of possibilities: Perhaps medical/genetic attributions are viewed these days as a kind of excuse for deviance. Number 2, a genetic attribution could signal that, "Look, those behavior patterns are part of the genes, they're permanent and unchangeable." Third, if threatening behavior is now believed to emanate from that individual's faulty genes, the observer may come to believe that the person really isn't fully human. Think of it this way: "I'm going to interact with this person, they are mentally ill and deviant, and it's because of their own DNA and genes. This person must be flawed to the very core of his or her being at the level of genotype."

A biogenetic model—especially if it's really reductionistic—could yield a view of the individual as permanently, unwaveringly flawed. This perspective could lead to subhumanization and could invoke the "tribal" exclusion module, over and above the other modules more typically related to mental illness of contagion or low social resources.

What's more accurate? As we emphasized throughout this course, it's that view of the mind—and of mental disorders—as a complex set of interactions and transactions between genes, biology, and experience. Perhaps such a view could be the ultimate defense against prejudice and stigma; but embracing this perspective is quite likely to require narratives, personal stories, and humanization, the subject of our next lecture.

Overall today, we've taken quite a momentous tour through evolutionary accounts of some of our most basic human tendencies: to be religious, to be aggressive rather than prosocial, and to show prejudice against and to stigmatize those in outgroups. I hope you agree that the perspective of evolution and natural selection can help us to understand how deeply ingrained some of these tendencies really are. Indeed, evolution has a major role in explaining social and cultural aspects of our minds.

Lecture Twenty-Three
Bringing in Personal Narratives

Scope:

Scientific knowledge about the mind and brain is rapidly accumulating, but much remains to be learned from narrative accounts of human experience. Human mythic skills reveal the essential nature of narrative. A vivid example is found in the fascinating yet harrowing story of the life of my father, a philosopher who began to experience severe symptoms of psychosis in adolescence, misdiagnosed as schizophrenia. A blend of risk factors and protective factors characterized his life. Only when I became a young adult did my father divulge the truth, going against medical advice, which led to a new diagnosis of bipolar disorder.

Outline

I. Science related to the human mind and human behavior has made great progress, but there is risk for its becoming an amalgamation of dry facts and findings unless it is balanced by narrative accounts of the life experiences of people who are subjects of research studies or who are treated for psychological distress.

II. A life narrative is a story of an individual's existence with a beginning, a middle, and an end. A host of such narratives have emerged in recent years, some that are first-person accounts and others that are sensitive and vivid case portrayals. These narratives help humanize mental and neurological disorders, and can reveal the potential for strength and resilience in our species.

   A. Indeed, humans are characterized by grammatical language and story-telling skills, revealing the mythic nature of our species, per Merlin Donald.

   B. Narrative places scientific variables and theories in a humanistic perspective.

   C. Contemplating and writing about personal experiences has additional benefits for the writer as well. Compared to writing equally-long passages about pleasant events or about neutral events, writing about negative events may help to prevent illnesses and to produce greater levels of psychological adjustment.

III. My father had a rich, troubled, and sometimes harrowing life; a brief account may be instructive with regard to humanizing severe mental illness.

    A. Born in 1919, Virgil Hinshaw Jr. was the youngest of 4 brothers; his mother was a missionary and his father was a Prohibitionist. His family history included both high achievement and cases of mood disorder, anxiety, and substance abuse.

    B. He lost his mother at age 3, and several years later, his stepmother engaged in a pattern of physical and sexual abuse. Even so, his childhood was marked by high academic achievement, athletic success, and a dedication to church.

    C. At age 16, in a period of mania, he jumped from the roof of the family home. For the next 6 months, he was chained to a bed in a public mental hospital. Still, without treatment, he recovered and went on to become high school valedictorian. His lasting diagnosis was schizophrenia, despite a clear pattern of repeated manic and depressive episodes.

    D. Despite academic success at Stanford and Princeton, and a budding career as a philosopher, he had additional, severe episodes.

    E. He became a professor at Ohio State, but his wife's pregnancies triggered serious episodes of mania and depression during the 1950s and 1960s.

    F. His doctors told him to "never tell your children about mental illness"—so the family was enshrouded in silence. In between episodes and absences, he was a generous and loving father.

    G. Only when I went away to college did my father begin to disclose his life's story. Not surprisingly, I gravitated toward psychology, the study of the mind, and toward work with children.

    H. I helped my father gain a correct diagnosis of bipolar disorder, 40 years after his initial episode.

IV. Near the end of my father's life, I wrote a narrative account of his life. This brief narrative raises several key themes and lessons.

    A. Accurate diagnosis of mental disorder is crucial in obtaining evidence-based treatment.

B. Both biological/genetic risk and life circumstances are necessary for mental disorder to emerge.

C. Resilience and courage are indeed possible in the face of serious risk.

D. Open discussion of family problems and secrets is essential— if done in ways that are sensitive to the age of the child—to prevent shame, silence, and internalization.

E. Disclosure and narrative can help to replace negative stereotypes with compassion, understanding, and a desire to learn more and develop effective treatment and rehabilitation programs.

F. Finding ways to reveal and share experiences may also be a key means of overcoming prejudice and stigma, opening all of us to the diversity and potential of the human species and the human mind.

V. My continuing goal is to blend rigorous science with humanizing personal and family narrative.

Suggested Reading:

Hinshaw, *Breaking the Silence.*

———, *The Years of Silence are Past.*

Jamison, *An Unquiet Mind.*

Questions to Consider:

1. Why might writing about or sharing one's personal narratives, particularly emotionally troubling ones, produce benefits to physical and emotional well being?

2. How can individuals with severe mental illness show strength, courage, and resilience, defying our stereotypes of mental disorder?

Lecture Twenty-Three—Transcript
Bringing in Personal Narratives

In our last lecture, we covered the evolutionary roots of 3 deep human tendencies: to be spiritual, to be aggressive, and to show prejudice. Today, our emphasis is on personal narratives and how they can play a key role in humanizing members of our species and in our overall understanding of the human mind. In other words, complementing everything else we've learned, your own personal and family experiences are also critical. Furthermore, as we'll learn, engaging in narratives could even be beneficial to your health.

To illustrate these points, I'm going to make some intensely personal disclosures of my family during this lecture. I hope that you find the material fascinating and illuminating; but at the same time, I'd like to forewarn you: Some of the narrative today is quite harrowing. But I tell it to you in the spirit of understanding the depths as well as the triumphs of the human spirit. My hope is that you might come away with a stance not unlike the distanced perspective that we will discuss: Not ignoring or denying painful narratives, but not becoming overly distressed, either; rather, emerging with a deeper perspective on what it means to be human.

The overall point is that without rich life narratives, our science of both individual development and the evolution of the human mind could become dry accumulations of facts. The goal today is to provide context and richness through personal and family narrative.

To introduce the narrative today, let's return to the 3 core views on human minds that we as a species have carried with us since we started recording our own histories: spirit-based views, naturalistic views, and humanistic views. I introduced these in our first lecture. Each of them plays a prominent role in today's narrative. Number 1: As you listen, think of how some of the "treatment"—and I really must put this term in quotes—my father received during his life was equivalent to care provided for wild animals, a pattern that has accompanied mental illness throughout history. On the other hand, his religious beliefs and his deeply spiritual nature were major guides and protective factors in his life. Number 2: My father often wondered throughout his life whether it might have been better if he had some physical disorder, even cancer; not a mental illness, which he inferred was "all in his mind." As we all grasp naturalistic accounts of mental illness better and better—that is, the genetic, physical, and brain-based realities that underlie serious mental disorder—we have to still understand that, at a different level of analysis, these disorders affect personal experience in a deep way.

Number 3, regarding humanistic views, my father's own career was as a philosopher, and a philosopher of science in particular, seeking to understand what is true. After being told flat out by his own doctors never to tell his children—my sister and me—about his lifelong bouts with mental illness, he finally gained the courage to go against medical advice once I started college and tell me over the next quarter century the narrative you're about to hear about his life's journey. In short, he himself embodied a humanistic, narrative approach in his own life. His recounting of his life narrative to me has now become my narrative for you.

In another sense, my dad's story reveals that to understand any life from a scientific and naturalistic perspective, it's vital to know the details of the individual case in all the richness and all of the despair that such details may provide as a counterpoint and as a complement to the formal research methods of naturalistic perspectives. Without personal, narrative details, we might not even know the right questions to ask in other more traditional forms of research.

Here's an important sidelight: Case reports and narratives are not valued terribly highly in most human science. Why? First, maybe the particular case isn't typical or representative; how much like other people with these particular risk factors or clinical features is this particular case? Second, how do we know if the variables provided in the narrative are the right ones? Many variables in a case study or narrative account remain uncontrolled; was this really the risk factor that the narrator thought it was, or was it actually another one, closely aligned with the first? Yet still, case studies, particularly those that bring in the person's unique perspectives, are truly crucial to understanding our minds and our minds' origins. A vivid case may help us to understand human experiences in ways that a quantitative study of correlations or risk factors never really can.

Here's another angle on this issue: Textbooks on research methods usually focus on how to verify what's true in nature; in testing hypotheses, we must use objective measures and exert careful control of extraneous variables, and replicate our findings. But what about the "discovery phase" of science; that is, deciding which hypotheses even to test in the first place? It may take deep understanding of the individual to get to the right factors and variables. For Darwin, certainly, it took a 5-year voyage on *The Beagle* around the world with his intense curiosity and study of rocks, plants, and animals to lay the foundation for evolutionary theory. In my own career, it took some real understanding of the seriousness of mental illness in my family before I could truly begin my pursuit of psychology and the origins of the human mind.

Finally, my dad's narrative points out quite vividly, I think, the strengths and accomplishments, and not just the sorrow and despair, which can accompany each mind's journey, even when mental disorder intercedes. I would like to convey this side of the coin, too.

What is, in fact, a narrative? It's the telling of a story; a temporal sequence of events. A life narrative, therefore, is a story of a person's development with a beginning, middle, and end, though not necessarily in that linear order. As Merlin Donald has emphasized, and as we have discussed in many lectures, humans are marked by mythic skills, involving explanations, sequential stories, causal accounts of the world around us, and the histories of who each of us is as a human. Think of stories around campfires, details of hunts, family lore to pass on to children, intense narratives about lineages and family trees; all of these are what make us human, creating our selves and our cultures. Indeed, we mark children's passage from the sensorimotor to the preoperational stage of cognitive development around the age of 2—remember Piaget from Lecture Nine—on the basis largely of symbolic, linguistic, narrative skills. In Merlin Donald's view, many modern human skills and abilities build upon humanity's mythic, narrative skills which subsequently, with the advent of written language and theoretical skills, have propelled abstraction and a deeper motivation to understand personal identity.

Consider this from current research: Contemplating and writing about personal experiences—in other words, creating narratives—has additional benefits for people who do so. The research of James Pennebaker, psychology professor at the University of Texas, reveals, in fact, substantial health benefits when people of different ages are asked to write about difficult emotional experiences. Through very careful experiments, those participants who are randomly assigned to write about struggles with difficult life events, compared to those who write equally-long passages about either pleasant events or neutral events, show lower rates of illness and higher rates of psychological adjustment subsequent to their narratives. It could well be that actively processing what has occurred in one's life, even if painful, is indeed necessary to work through it.

Research from Ozlem Ayduk, a personality psychologist and my colleague at UC Berkeley, reveals hints about some of the optimal ways to do such processing of negative experiences. Rather than ignoring or denying the events altogether—or rather, too, than becoming embroiled in them and inflamed by them—gaining a "cool," third-person distance perspective could be optimal for adjustment. In other words, being able to process the events from this somewhat-distanced vantage point appears to be beneficial. It's easier said than done; there's some controversy about how best to make it happen. In the history of therapy, psychodynamic views have emphasized deep, time-consuming processes of emotionally working through unconscious material. Cognitive behavioral therapies, on the other hand, tend to utilize through a present focus specific cognitive exercises. Newer approaches add emotion back into these cognitive strategies, fostering means of regulating and gaining perspective on the often intense affect that can accompany major life stresses and problems. All forms of psychotherapy and of social support more generally try to provide us tools to engage in emotional meaning and insight, but to disengage from counterproductive emotional rumination or dysregulation. The key question is how to gain such perspective. Narrative may be one path.

Now for my own family and personal narrative; there's a lot of richness here, and I can present only a small part of the detail. My father, named Virgil Hinshaw Jr., was born in 1919. He was the fourth of 4 brothers, born to a missionary mother and a Prohibitionist father, Virgil Sr., just outside of Chicago. His relatives included many with high achievement, but also a good number with mood disorder, anxiety problems, substance abuse, and eating disorders in some of the women of the family. Here's a big key risk factor in my dad's life: His mother died rather suddenly when he was 3 years of age in surgery for a tumor. We know that losing a parent before the age of 5 is indeed a risk factor for later mood disorders, but we also know today that it's really the quality of the subsequent caregiving that actually has stronger effects, potentially serving as a protective factor.

What of my father's brothers? They were indeed the motherless Hinshaw boys, as shown in a photo in a national Prohibition newsletter in 1923. My uncle Harold was the oldest, at this point a preteen, who later had serious problems with alcoholism. Next in order of age was my uncle Randall, who became an economist, who was extremely supportive of my dad during and after his episodes. Third was my uncle Robert, who became dedicated to a career in both psychology and psychiatry after witnessing my father's first psychotic episode and suicide attempt. However, with his medical license, he began to self-administer pain medications, and became addicted. Then, fourth, was my father: Junior, as he was called, Virgil Jr.

Subsequently my grandfather remarried, also to a missionary, and they settled out west in Pasadena, California. Two more boys emerged from this new union. My dad's stepmother was proud of his academic and athletic skills and accomplishments, and his religious training, but she singled him out among the 4 original boys for very harsh punishments. She treated him, in fact, as she had some of the girls at missionary schools during her earlier career. At times, my dad had to wait for hours to receive a switching. Later there was a decidedly sexualized flavor to the punishments, as she rubbed in oils to help heal the wounds toward his adolescent years. As my father wrote years later in his journals, "I was the victim of what today we might call child abuse." But at the time, there was silence; no one else in the family knew, and my father did not disclose. All too often, this is the pattern with abusive experiences.

We know today that abuse is not the primary cause of bipolar disorder, but we also know that it may interact with the genetic predisposition for bipolar disorder to make for a particularly difficult course of this illness. Indeed, we have discussed extensively throughout this course that in terms of individual development, it's typically combinations of risk factors that tend to produce the worst outcomes.

Throughout his childhood and adolescence, my father continued with his academic and athletic pursuits; and he had a wit, maybe even some oppositionality from an early age. In first grade, for example, a substitute teacher tried to discipline the increasingly disruptive class. My father was challenged by this teacher about his attitude. "Well," he said, climbing on top of a desk, "if you don't like my attitude, how about my altitude?" Harsh punishment awaited him at home, when the principal let the family know. Overall, however, he studied hard, attended church, and played sports, with football and shot-putting his 2 favorite sporting events.

When he was 16, in the mid-1930s, my dad became preoccupied with world fascism. Visitors to the family home—part of the international prohibition movement—had, in the preceding years, warned my grandfather, my dad, and his brothers at the family dinner table of the coming of Hitler and Mussolini in Europe. In 1936—and with hindsight, I can now say this was a developing manic episode, not known at the time—after several days of sleeplessness, my father jumped from the roof of the family home (just a 1-story bungalow, fortunately), believing 2 things: That he could fly, and that this flight would convince world leaders to stop Hitler and Mussolini. Clearly, he had developed delusions by this point.

For the next 6 months, he was chained to his bed in a public mental hospital. At one point several months later, my grandfather was called in by the superintendent: His beloved son Junior had gone from 180 pounds to 120 pounds, delusionally believing now that the food at the hospital was poisoned. He had experienced a severe manic episode, going from stage 1 to 2 to 3, followed by a devastating mixed state; but the lasting diagnosis at the time was schizophrenia, following the trend of American diagnostic practices.

Somehow, without any treatment—no medication, no therapy—he recovered 6 months later and went on to become high school valedictorian. We know now that in some cases of bipolar disorder, almost complete recovery between episodes occurs. But, think of his religious faith that had helped him during his hospitalization; and his love of learning, and his intensive study habits, kicked back in as soon as he was out. Through some combination of reasons, he was himself again.

Despite academic success—considerable success—at Stanford and then at Princeton, where, as a graduate student, he studied both with Bertrand Russell and Albert Einstein, and a budding career as a philosopher, my father had additional, severe experiences, including a stay at Philadelphia State Hospital after the completion of his Ph.D. in Philosophy. During his half-year stay in 1945, not long after he had completed his doctoral dissertation, he became convinced that he was being held in a concentration camp in Europe, as revealed to me by my uncle Randall after he had taken my father on a day pass drive outside the facility, during which my father had translated the road signs immediately into German. This again was a clear delusion; but note that Hitler's goals were to rid the world not only of Jews, but gays and lesbians, Gypsies, and those with mental retardation and mental illness.

As I learned a few years ago in researching a book I wrote about the stigmatization of mental illness, Philadelphia State Hospital was known at the time as the worst mental hospital in the United States—it was, in fact, the subject of the book and film *The Snake Pit*—with the men's dorm, especially, looking eerily like the multiple bunks of the concentration camps in Europe. My father's belief was, in fact, delusional; but there was a germ of truth and recognition in it.

He recovered again. He became a professor of philosophy at Ohio State, where he met my mother, a graduate student in history. They fell in love and got married. But during my mother's pregnancies with me and then my sister in the 1950s, there were serious episodes of mania and depression in my dad. He was treated in 1954 with the first antipsychotic medication, Thorazine, maybe the fourth patient in the United States to receive it. He also received numerous ECTs, electroconvulsive therapies, or shock treatment. When performed today, these can be a very effective treatment for some forms of severe depression, but it was often not well-delivered back then.

His doctors told him "Never tell your children about mental illness, they can't understand"; so the young family was enshrouded in silence, even during the entire year, when I was in third grade, that my father was hospitalized back in California. In between episodes and absences, my dad was generous and loving. During one spring break, the young family played shuffleboard together in Florida. When my dad was present, he helped me to understand hard problems, and he was kind and understanding when I was afraid. Once, when I was in kindergarten, and he was home between episodes, I had a burning question for him: how Russia could be the biggest country in area but China had more people. I dared to ask him whether China might actually have 100 more people than Russia. My father's response was kind and sincere: "This will be hard to believe, son, but there are actually more than 100 more people in China than in Russia!" I'll really never forget his patience.

In fourth grade, sleepless and afraid, I called out, saying that I might die one night; this is the year after he had been gone for nearly 12 months. My father awoke to come into my bedroom and comfort me and tell me that I might live to be 100 years old, in fact, with the miracles of modern medicine; that magical number of 100 was soothing. Maybe he, in fact, wondered whether any such advances or miracles could help him.

Overall, individuals, even with severe mental illness, can be, indeed, sensitive parents. Only when I went away to college did my dad begin to disclose his life's story to me, during spring breaks and winter vacations home. These were hard talks, for sure, but I realized instantly that they were the truth. Naturally enough, I became interested in psychology; and clinical psychology in particular. I also gravitated toward work with children in high risk situations, and those with mental and developmental disorders.

My dad's revelations did not come without anxiety for me, about my own risk for mental illness. But as we discussed in Lecture Twenty-One, there could well be an adaptive advantage when an individual carries a partial genetic loading for mental disorder, bipolar disorder in particular. Perhaps I have benefitted from some of the energy and sensitivity but not the full force of the manic-depressive spectrum.

After graduating from college, I helped to get my dad a correct diagnosis of bipolar disorder—40 years after his initial episode—in 1976. His latter years were marked by a gradual and then more precipitous cognitive decline; whether from the untreated episodes or from the effects of the wrong treatments he'd been receiving is not clear. But I opened up enough to ask his permission in some of our last talks together to write about and talk about his life. My dad still looked pretty vibrant into his 60s, but he had become frail in his early 70s. I did end up writing about his life, completing the work after his death in 1995 from a Parkinson-like illness, which again could have originated from the years of untreated and maltreated mental disorder.

A narrative of a parent is often linked to the narrative of the offspring. My own childhood was marked by anxiety and control, and lots of sports and lots of studying back in the Midwest. In fact, I have very few memories of my father's departures and returns, given the strict code of family silence prescribed by his doctors. In college, despite my fascination and interest in learning my dad's life, I really had intense reactions. I myself was afraid of losing control and perhaps going to a mental hospital, especially if I couldn't sleep at night. But at the same time, as I noted, I was greatly drawn to working with children, and to learning about the mind; its powers and its disorders. I gradually realized that telling my dad's and my own story could help me to understand why I care about the science of the mind, and why the integration of personal, scientific, and clinical is really the ultimate goal.

This narrative—all too brief—I think raises several key themes and lessons. Number 1: Accurate diagnosis of mental disorder is absolutely crucial in obtaining evidence-based treatment. Let's play devil's advocate: Maybe diagnosis didn't really matter a half century ago or more, when treatments were nonexistent or primitive. My dad would in all likely have been chained to his bed in the 1930s regardless of a diagnosis of schizophrenia, bipolar disorder, or anything else. But today, and increasingly in the future, accurate diagnosis may make a major difference for responsive treatment.

Number 2: Biological and genetic risk and life circumstances are necessary for mental disorder to emerge. This has been a key theme throughout the course. Consider my dad's family history; it clearly includes some genetic vulnerability for mood disorder and other mental illnesses. But consider, too, his early experiences: loss of his mother at 3, his experiences of abuse. Again, interactive and transactional models are where the action is.

Third: Resilience and courage are clearly possible, even in the face of serious life risk and mental illness. How did he return from 6 months in a back ward to become valedictorian? Bipolar disorder, unlike some other forms of mental illness, is linked to achievement and success; but it's a mistake to romanticize the "highs" of hypomania, which, as we've discussed, all too often progress into Stages Two and Three, leading to destruction. Again, despite the stereotypes, my dad was quite warm and sensitive to me. He kept teaching and kept performing his research despite devastating hospitalizations. But without the tenure system, perhaps he would never have kept his job. His humor, his deeply philosophical attitude—indeed, in the last years of his life, he told me that he wouldn't have traded any of his life experiences, even the psychoses and hospitalizations—his religious beliefs, his faith in science; all of these, I'm sure, played a role. Perhaps, too, some of his genes gave him the predisposition to a form of bipolar disorder with a strong return to normal functioning in between episodes.

Here's a fourth point: Open discussion of family problems and secrets is really essential, if they are done in ways that are sensitive to the age and needs of the child to prevent shame, silence, and internalization. In fact, it was my mother who had to endure the worst of the episodes, largely in silence herself. She was the unsung hero who kept the whole family together, so often the case when family members must rally. But what should my mother and father have told my sister and me? It's really hard to imagine, given the utter silence that was prescribed and followed. I think any words would have been better than enforced silence, which too often leads children to internalize and blame themselves.

Here's an important clinical revelation: William Beardslee, at Harvard Medical School, has devised a particular form of family therapy specifically in cases where one or both parents has a mood disorder. The main feature of this therapy involves creating a narrative to tell the child; so the family works with the therapist in child-friendly terms to describe dad's episodes, mom's moodiness, etc. This treatment reduces stress, facilitates coping, and may actually prevent the onset of mood disorders in the child some years later as he or she matures. Narrative, mind you, is the key to this therapy, outweighing even genetic risk in helping to stop the intergenerational pattern of mood disorders.

Here's a fifth point: Disclosure and narrative can, I believe, help to replace negative stereotypes with compassion, understanding, and a desire to learn more and to develop better, effective treatment and rehabilitation programs. By understanding the realities and not just the stereotypes of mental illness, we may be able to engage public discussion and force the issue of the sheer numbers of individuals whose minds have gone awry. This fifth point about narrative is number 5 on my list, but it could have been first; because, in fact, if there had been more openness and disclosure back in the 1930s, maybe my dad would have been able to get a more accurate diagnosis earlier (of course, if the field had been more sophisticated as well).

I must disclose this: One of my own struggles as a scientist has been how to blend naturalism and science on the one hand with narrative and expressive methods on the other. Many responses from audiences and students to my telling of this narrative have been quite revealing to me; people have told me they didn't believe it was possible, for example, in the scientific study of the mind to have any room for personal experience and narrative. Others have commented on their fascination that the personal and historical could actually lead to a deeper appreciation of science. In sum, this integration in my life and career, though not easy to come by, has been richly rewarding.

Thank you for listening to my own, and my father's, narrative. Finding ways to reveal and share experiences may be the key means of overcoming prejudice and stigma, opening all of us to the diversity and potential of the human species, the human mind, and our full human capacities. Considering your own experiences could clue you in to the origins of your own minds at some level. You could do this via writing, talking, seeking support, or, more generally, expressing both difficult and positive experiences.

The point is this: Experiences can help to foster coping, so long as we don't dwell entirely on the negative but work to overcome it. Narrative can help to make sense of our lives, and may help us to understand the humanity deep inside all of us. After all, narrative is the quality and skill that is one of the true essences of our species.

Lecture Twenty-Four
The Future of the Human Mind

Scope:

This course has attempted to integrate individual development and evolutionary development—a daunting task, given our still imperfect knowledge of both domains. Among the many frontier areas in the study of the mind, we discuss renewed interest in unconscious mental processes; the exponential growth of computers and artificial intelligence; advances in the study of consciousness; mind engineering; and applications of scientific findings to key social problems. The study of the mind has the potential to foster the development of positive as well as negative human attributes; whether our species' heightened awareness of brains and minds can fuel a healthier and more humane world remains to be seen. Overall, sciences of the mind and humanities require further integration.

Outline

I. This course has provided a tour of the origins of the human mind at 2 levels: on an evolutionary scale and through each individual's developmental path.

II. What will the continued study of the human mind entail in terms of new frontiers? It is hard to provide valid guesses given the fast pace of progress; but the following are leading contenders.

   A. Many more mental and emotional processes take place at unconscious levels than previously thought.

   B. Artificial intelligence and the growth of computers could either enhance our well-being or threaten the existence and viability of the human mind.

   C. The study of human consciousness is now a viable area of investigation.

   D. The ever-growing potential for us to engineer our own minds, and our own evolution, is one of the greatest and most controversial frontiers for our species.

   F. The linking of the mind with broad social issues is another key frontier.

III. Will future investigations of the mind be used for good or for ill?

    A. The same question has been asked about physics, with respect to our understanding of the nature of the atom and of the universe; about genetics and genomics, with respect to engineering our own life blueprints, DNA; and about the inner workings of our unique human consciousness.

    B. Perhaps the key question is how to maintain ethical control over our ever-changing discoveries related to the science of the brain and mind, including the emerging field of neuroethics.

IV. Overall, a fundamental dualism between objective, naturalistic accounts of the mind and subjective, narrative portrayals reveals a key tension in the sciences and humanities.

Suggested Reading:

Hawkins and Blakeslee, *On Intelligence.*

Kurzweil, *The Singularity Is Near.*

Questions to Consider:

1. With the very real potential for super-intelligent computers and for intentionally directing our own evolution through genetic manipulation, what will it mean in the future to be human?

2. What is your list of the key issues that will confront those interested in the human mind in the coming years?

Lecture Twenty-Four—Transcript
The Future of the Human Mind

This course has provided a tour of the origins of the human mind at 2 levels: First, on an evolutionary scale, across hundreds of millions of years, extending even to several billion years if we include the earliest life forms; and second, through each individual's developmental path across the decades of a human life. A fair question is this: Have we succeeded in completely integrating these 2 perspectives? Well, to be honest, not entirely; given that our knowledge of the underlying processes of each is still so incomplete. We still don't know some basic principles of genes and evolution. The fossil records of some of the earliest animals, over 500 million years ago, are incomplete; and the fossil records hominid brains and behaviors can never be complete, as brains and behaviors don't leave fossils. What a mystery, still, to understand how each human brain and mind forms across the earliest weeks, months, and years of life, with the billions of neurons and trillions of synapses that form, guided by processes that are still far from completely understood.

But we are getting ever closer to understanding how evolution and development interact. We now know, for example, that evolution has shaped particular genes, which ultimately result in our species in enormous plasticity and learning, because our status as a species that learns, and learns a lot, led to great reproductive success.

Evolution has prepared our species for long periods of individual development and long periods of initial helplessness. These, in turn, have created the need for intense emotional bonds between caregivers and offspring, with the lifelong emotional implications of our earliest attachments. Evolution has also shaped our executive functions, our abilities to understand and regulate our emotions—though far from completely, as we all know when we lose our temper or fail to act as we should when we're fearful—and to negotiate intensely complex social and cultural lives we all have. Natural selection has created in us a broad potential for culture, invention, entire institutions devoted to education, and the means, recently, of intentionally directing our own evolution, through our huge increase in knowledge of genes and some basic facts about how we evolved; and both individual development and natural selection operate through complex interactions of biology and environmental contexts.

Overall, in many ways, the origins of our minds via evolution and the origins of each mind during individual development are quite closely linked, and the science related to this integration is increasing in sophistication and power each year. Our topics throughout the course have been wide-ranging: Of course, evolution and natural selection have been core topics; microevolution, in fact, contains some of the most exciting science today. But we also considered advances in psychological theories of minds, from psychodynamic and social learning views to the cognitive and emotion revolutions of the later 20th century and beyond.

The key stages of the human lifespan, as we emphasized, are temperament and attachment in infancy; family, socialization and stages of cognitive development in childhood; executive functions, emotion regulation, and identity in adolescence; and altered time perspectives, positive bias, and wisdom as we age. At the same time, we dealt extensively with the ways in which genes and biology on the one hand, and experience on the other, interact and transact. The term "nature versus nurture" may never emanate from your lips again; or if so, only with full appreciation of the combinations of nature and nurture that shape our development.

We spent a great deal of time on connections between the great human potential in each of our minds and human limitations and pathology, and how the 2 are so closely intertwined; the study of one truly facilitates the study of the other.

Returning to evolution, we learned that principles of natural selection can help us understand how mental illness, despite its genetic roots and its devastating impairments, has persisted throughout human history. Evolution also helps to explain religious tendencies, propensities to be aggressive, and our widespread tendencies to show prejudice toward humans who are different from ourselves.

Throughout, we emphasized personal narratives and how these could be a key means of emphasizing human individuality. Our mythic, linguistic, story-telling skills emerged during our transition to humanity as a species, and are still one of the crowning products of our species' evolution, along with others we've discussed: time travel, inhibitory control, mental synthesis, and emotion regulation. The transition a few thousand years ago to theoretical, written skills is, of course, another huge advance, not least in the abilities of our minds to reflect upon and even improve themselves.

Throughout the course, all of these issues and themes have betrayed 2 perspectives: one that is quite powerful and optimistic, and another that is far more sobering and pessimistic. On the optimistic side, the mind is unprecedented in its power and potential. But at the same time, our species tends to recreate, in nearly any new environment in which it finds itself, core tendencies to dominate other species, use up core resources on our planet, castigate members of outgroups, and commit high rates of within-species violence, even genocide; and experience, generation after generation, debilitating mental disorders, which, as we stated, reflect a mismatch between our genetic heritage and our current environments. It's clear that our species hasn't yet solved some core problems of our existence.

Our emphasis today is on what the future study of the human mind may entail and reveal, and, indeed, on what future minds may look like as well. Let's consider some key frontiers: We'll start with the unconscious. We've discussed previously that many more mental and emotional processes take place at an unconscious level than we previously thought; the evolutionary psychology perspective, in fact, contends that our minds are composed of a host of relatively specific modules, each shaped by natural selection to solve problems our species had to contend with. The unconscious mind uncovered by today's science looks quite different from the cauldrons of instinctive sexual and aggressive energy in Freudian terms. Current terminology emphasizes what we call "implicit" processes, those that exist below conscious awareness. Let's look at some examples.

First: our implicit attitudes; those that exist below awareness but can still lead to fascinating behavioral responses. One way to test this is to "prime" subjects in research studies. "Primes" are prompts or cues, but masked ones; the research participant doesn't realize the intent of the researcher. An investigator might give word lists to be remembered, including certain terms that may color the person's underlying attitudes. The researcher doesn't really care if the person learns the words very well, but that's the cover story so that the subject doesn't know the real point of the investigation, to be influenced by the primes. Here's an example; fascinating research from John Bargh, the eminent social psychologist from Yale. His team primed subjects with words that might be associated with aging. For example, in word lists, there were the terms "Florida," or "sentimental," or "wrinkle," but no direct mention of elderly people. After this priming, the research subjects in that condition walk slower in the hallway later on during the experiment, and even forget more about what they did than those primed with other words. Something was clearly happening at an unconscious level regarding attitudes and corresponding behaviors. All of us may well have underlying mental scripts or schemas that exist below everyday awareness.

After implicit attitudes, we can consider implicit perception. Let's get right to an incredible study that emerged in late 2008; it gave more credence to the process called "blindsight," the ability to see without even knowing that we are seeing. Here, in this case, a doctor in his 50s had become completely blind through several terrible strokes that had blocked key areas of the visual cortex in the occipital lobe from receiving sufficient blood; so his visual centers could not process visual stimuli from the retina any longer. To help science, he allowed himself—although he was initially hesitant—to be examined as he navigated a very difficult obstacle course. Here's what noted science writer Ben Carey of the *New York Times* wrote:

When he finally tried it, though, something remarkable happened: He zigzagged down the hall, sidestepping a garbage can, a tripod, a stack of paper, and several boxes as if he could see everything clearly. A researcher shadowed him in case he stumbled. ... The study, which included extensive brain imaging, is the most dramatic demonstration to date of so-called blindsight, the native ability to sense things using the brain's primitive, subcortical—and entirely subconscious—visual system.

This was the first demonstration of blindsight in a person whose visual centers in the occipital lobes had been completely destroyed. What happened? First, this man did have use of his eyes and a healthy brain until the time of the strokes; so he did have a history of receiving visual input. But second, we know that visual signals go through 2 key circuits: first, from the retina to the visual cortex in the occipital lobe—but in his case, that had been destroyed—and second, from the retina to the superior colliculus and even the amygdala, structures subcortical, well below the cortex, that can process visual information without conscious awareness or any visual image that gets recorded in the brain. Even without the brain regions typically associated with vision, a more primitive, subcortical brain circuit utilized visual signals without any awareness on the participant's part to navigate the obstacle course.

Here's something even more intriguing: This same doctor showed what we call "emotional blindsight," meaning that when he was presented with photos of threatening faces, he cringed automatically, as do other people, even though he could not actually "see" the faces. This secondary, unconscious, implicit visual system registers both solid objects and social signals, like faces, but without any conscious awareness of having "seen" them. There are great potentials here for rehabilitation, if we could somehow teach people with "conscious" impairments of perception to utilize this older, more intuitive brain system, which is usually bypassed with our more sophisticated systems in place.

Third on our tour is implicit memory: We can actually "remember" things we have learned without any conscious awareness. There's a host of examples: At an everyday level, shoe tying, once it becomes automatized, is actually harmed by thinking too hard about doing it, trying to remember it; once a skill is automatized, it is sort of refractory to conscious awareness. Infants prefer their mothers' voices at very young ages—a month or 2—over other voices saying the same words, showing that they remember hearing those maternal voices from the time that they were in utero, but without any conscious awareness.

Finally, even those high-level aspects of thought—like language and complex problem solving—rely on a large number of complex, unconscious algorithms of parallel-processed modular mental programs; there's a bevy of instinctual programs in our minds with which were born and which we develop in our first years of life.

Overall, it's clear: Many key processes of the human mind operate without conscious awareness by the "operator"; that is, the individual in question. We're certain to hear more about such developments and discoveries with respect to our minds' unconscious programs in the years ahead; and as just noted, there could be incredible potential for rehabilitation if unconscious perception could be harnessed.

From the unconscious mind, let's move to unconscious machinery—computers—and whether they might actually become conscious.

We're going to tour briefly artificial intelligence and the growth of computers, which could either further enhance our well-being or in some views threaten the existence of the human mind and species. Let's being with an important "test" devised in the middle of the 20th century: The mathematician Alan Turing proposed that artificial intelligence will truly have come of age when the following occurs: You sit down and have a "talk" with a computer and a parallel talk with another human being, and you can't tell the difference. No computer, even as powerful as some computers are now, can yet pass the Turing Test; but how soon?

With regard to this, in 1965 Gordon Moore, the founder of Intel, proposed that there would be an exponential growth in the number of transistors on integrated circuits. He's been dead-on for the last 45 years or so; computer circuitry has shown this exponential curve. There may be limits at some point as the size scale of nanotubes and electron-level processing is getting fast approached. But extending this model, some have proposed that hard drive capacity, and by extension computer "intelligence," will double every 2 years as well.

In terms of predictions, Ray Kurzweil, an inventor and futurist whose predictions have sometimes been borne out—he's also a discoverer of voice recognition software, symphonic music synthesizers, and much else—is a proponent of what he calls "transhumanism." He believes that humanity's future is related to an exponential expansion of knowledge, taking Moore's Law into what he calls a "Law of Accelerating Returns." His claim is this: Our biological evolution is on the verge of being superseded not only by cultural evolution, as we've discussed, across the past several thousand years, but currently by a radical technological evolution, through we're going to be able to manipulate our minds through self-aware, self-organizing machine intelligence. Supercomputers, in this view, will be able to apply complex programs to their own hardware and software, eventually leaving the human mind quite far behind. Brain-computer interfaces, beyond what we currently have, and even "advanced computer programs" that could be loaded into our brains could actually take place.

Kurzweil predicts that late in the 21st century, the "singularity" will occur, when the Turing Test will be passed. Machine intelligence and human interface will be so advanced that technology, the entire world situation, and our definition of humanity will radically change. The new computers will recognize humans at that point as their ancestors. The human mind will seem rather pedestrian and unskilled in the face of such computing power. Yet some other scientists and visionaries are not at all convinced by this kind of prediction: Jeff Hawkins, inventor of the Palm Pilot and active promoter of computational neuroscience, believes that no truly artificial, machine intelligence can go that far, unless it could be grounded in a body. In other words, our brains and minds "work" only because they are bound in bones, muscles, and emotions; they operate through perceiving a world actively and experiencing it through behavior. They can't truly function in a disembodied state. It takes social and emotional inputs to enable our computing and predicting brains, and our neocortex, to truly make sense of the world and solve problems. Our minds work the way they do, according to Hawkins, because of their means of detecting patterns and making predictions beyond computations per se. But this can't happen without the entire context of social connections, emotions, and the senses we experience.

Does this bring to mind our earlier discussions of dualism? I think it should. Perhaps there is no such thing as a mind that is completely disconnected from a body (despite those cartoons of mad scientists creating brains in vats and beakers, with fumes and electric currents feeding the liquids in which the brains are suspended). Overall, the future of the human mind, and of artificial minds, is a hot topic indeed, with definitions of humanity, dualism, and morality at the forefront.

Third, regardless of whether machines will become more fully conscious, our minds are; so the study of human consciousness is now front and center in the study of the mind. As we discussed, for decades dismissed as speculative and nonscientific, investigations of human consciousness—that is, how we display our apparently unique ability to reflect on our own behavior; plan for our envisioned futures; experience the sense of colors, memories, and perceptions; and create intricate personal narratives—are now proliferating as one of the key areas in all of cognitive science. Certainly, many of our mental modules are unconscious, as we just discussed; but something is occurring that facilitates our self-awareness, our meta-awareness—in other words, our awareness of our awareness—and our active sense of the future and our ability to plan for it.

Some scientists and philosophers have contended that it might actually take a kind of "theory of relativity" of the brain and mind—something outside the ways we construe our brain chemistry and ourselves, in the way that Einstein connected time and gravity to our usual conceptions of space—to comprehend finally how our billions of neurons and nearly uncountable numbers of synaptic interconnections could produce the ineffable and profound self-perceptions and "flavor of life" that our consciousness entails. Perhaps this remains an enigma because our minds were "constructed" by natural selection to do a variety of human tasks, but—as Steven Pinker reminds us—these tasks did not include understanding their own nature, at least not very easily.

Next, a fourth frontier: the ever-growing potential for us to engineer our own brain and minds; this is one of the greatest and most controversial issues our species now faces. We covered a bit of this ground a few moments ago in discussing the growth of supercomputers; but on another front, gene therapies are beginning to exist now for certain devastating neurological disorders like Duchenne muscular dystrophy, which is a single-gene disease. On the other side, however, we have to consider the potential for good and evil regarding the detection of high-risk fetuses; for example, those who carry genes that may confer risk for mental disorder. As we discussed in Lecture Eighteen, we could be cutting down greatly on the genetic diversity of our species if we embark upon unthinking detection and prevention practices, especially related to mood disorders and bipolar disorder. The implications here for who we are as a species are profound.

Further study of the plasticity of the human mind and the plasticity in each brain is quite essential; it will place priority on discovering the kinds of environments that can maximize human potential and help the brain to literally rewire itself.

Finally, the mind and its study are clearly linked with broad social issues. Understanding the mind better should help us to be able to deal with such core issues as climate change, the gross disparities in income across the nation and indeed the world, and population control. These are issues traditionally linked to political science, environmental science, and other fields, but if we can understand better not only how our minds evolved but how they currently configure risk, understand social problems and the state of the world, social and political policies may have a far better chance of actually working. It's going to take a large mass of efforts spanning computer science, ethics, politics, history, neuroscience, human development, anthropology, and many more fields to be able to integrate our sense of our minds' purely cognitive, computational abilities with our sense of compassion, social justice, and planning for the Earth's future.

As a summary question: Will future investigations of the mind, and future endeavors along the lines of "mind control," be used for good or for ill? The same question, of course, has been—and will continue to be—asked about physics, with respect to our understanding of the nature of the atom and nucleus, with direct implications for the construction of atomic and nuclear bombs; and it has clearly been asked about genetics and genomics, with respect to engineering our own life blueprints (that is, our DNA). Maybe the key question will be how to develop better understanding of ethics, including the evolution of our development of ethical principles, and how and in what ways ethics can and should guide our scientific efforts.

In fact, the field neuroethics has come into its own recently, addressing a host of relevant questions. There are 2 main subdivisions of neuroethics: first, what's called the "ethics of neuroscience"; for example, what are the implications of brain imaging, brain implants, and computer-human interface for the good of our species? Then the counterpoint: the neuroscience of ethics; in other words, what brain regions and processes are likely to be involved in ethical principles and ethical decision-making in all humans? With regard to the first, there are big questions about the difference between treating a brain-based disorder with medications or implants or other neuro-related methods and enhancing normal functioning by such means. For example, can all of us—not just those with ADHD—do better cognitively with stimulant medications, or other neuro-enhancing medications still under development? A basic response from me is caveat emptor; far more needs to be learned about any such general enhancement strategies.

E. O. Wilson in his book *Consilience*, asserts this: The arts, humanities, ethics, and natural sciences can truly come together and achieve a true unification; that's the meaning of the word "concilience." This is a bold prediction, given the traditional rifts between ethics and justice, the humanistic tradition, and naturalistic, brain-based perspectives.

Here's one thought, at least, along these lines: Whatever the sophistication of our future scientific and genetic advances, what will continue to mark us as a species is our mythic skills: our storytelling abilities, our making sense of our selves and our lives through narratives. What marks us as well is our intense desire to understand our own natures. This desire brings us back to another take on dualism: Are purely scientific explanations of thoughts, emotions, executive functions, time travel, and other mental skills ever going to be completely satisfactory? I think it's doubtful, because we realize inside us that there is a difference in "level of analysis" between, on the one hand, a biochemical/neurotransmitter-based explanation of how our minds might work the way they do, or a natural-selection explanation as to how a particular mental module evolved; and, on other hand, the content and feeling of that particular mental or emotional function. Stories and narratives will still continue to play a key role on the experiential side.

The only certainties in the future may well be the following: The quick pace of future discoveries, particularly related to a new evolutionary direction for our species; and the lag between such efforts and our species' ability to link human values and ethics with the optimal utilization of these kinds of discoveries. A core question from this course is whether scientists of the future will be able to get ever closer to understanding the specific evolutionary origins of the human mind. We still don't know just which genes, and when they were selected, and how they were expressed, really gave our species, for example, spoken, flexible, and grammatical language. When this course is taught in 50 years, there may be a whole lot more specific information to impart. It's going to take many disciplines, converging in their efforts, to elucidate key evolutionary principles related to our minds' true origins.

In closing, let me give one suggestion and one wish, if I may. Here's the suggestion: Given what we know about individual development, we might enhance human potential by providing young children with a whole lot of opportunity to play in stimulating but relatively simple environments—this has been aptly suggested by my Berkeley colleague, developmental psychologist Alison Gopnik, among many others—rather than a premature rush to academic readiness at age 1, 2, or 3. Human children learn through rich opportunities to play, not through rote, uncreative curricula before their minds are really ready.

Now, the wish: Could be granted just one day—maybe even just a few hours—every century or so, to come back and get a brief update on the future of our species' investigations of the origins of the human mind? Is that really too much to ask? What a treat it would be. But come to think of it, I might want to advance that schedule from every century to every 20 or 40 years, given the fast pace of current and undoubtedly future advances.

I want thank each of you for participating in this course, which I've enjoyed immensely. Above all, I hope that you gained some appreciation of the interlinking of evolution, individual development, the intensely social nature of our species, and the need to humanize rather than castigate our human diversity. We are truly at a crossroads with respect to our future, given the real problems of crowding, food, ethnic strife, our increasingly toxic planet, and the clash between our early-human brains and minds and today's major social and personal problems. There's a continuing dualism between objective, naturalistic accounts of the mind and subjective, narrative portrayals. This rift reveals a fundamental tension between the sciences and humanities. As we grope to understand the ultimate origins of the human mind, both perspectives are going to remain vital.

I do believe this: More knowledge, more understanding, and more compassion are our main hopes for the future as we continue to probe the ultimate origins of the human mind.

Again, thank you. I hope that your own minds have been stretched and challenged though our examination of the origins and development of the human mind.

Timelines

A. Integrative Timeline of Prehuman and Human History

Part I: Prehuman History

Key:　Ma = Millions of years ago
　　　 Ka = Thousands of years ago
　　　 Ya = Years ago

Note: Entries in bold are not directly on the "path" to modern humans. They are included to reveal patterns of convergent evolution in different evolutionary trajectories, during natural selection.

Time	Species	Neuronal/ brain Features	Some functional capacities
590 Ma	jellyfish	While no brain, neurons form in epidermis in a "nerve net."	Basic sensation and motor response.
550 Ma	segmented worms	Brain consisting of ganglia and cords, with giant axons; some have rudimentary forebrain, midbrain, and hindbrain.	Detection of light, chemicals, and contact; withdrawal of body from danger.
525 Ma	vertebrates	All house brain inside cranium with brainstem; even early vertebrates have forebrain, midbrain, hindbrain; neurogenesis, synaptogenesis, and some myelination occur	Regulation of body functions, sexual behavior, and locomotion.
400 Ma	**insects**	Brains with capability for perceiving sounds and scents; neurogenesis, synaptogenesis, and myelination occur.	Flying, highly organized societal structures in some species; perception of social "dance" signals in honeybees.

375–450 Ma	jawed vertebrates	Greatly increased myelination.	Faster neural transmission; able to eat larger prey, with increased energy stores.
325 Ma	reptiles	Limbic system.	Rage, fight-flight responses.
180 Ma	mammals	Neocortex, 6-layered dorsal region.	Social bonds, rudimentary problem solving, and better memory.
150 Ma	**birds**	Well-developed cerebellum and visual system.	Some species begin learning song and memory of migration routes; dimorphisms in brain, seen relating to male song patterns
120 Ma	placental mammals	A wider pelvic opening in females allows the birth of young with larger brains.	Enhanced problem-solving.
55–65 Ma	primates	Enhanced cerebellum, thicker cortex, and a larger brain.	Motor coordination; stereoscopic vision; and single births, leading to a slower period of individual development.
20 Ma	upright primates	Larger frontal cortex.	Bidepalism, more intensive social bonds, and more use of opposable thumb.

*Note: Hominid separation from lineage with chimpanzees: 5–7 Ma.

7 Ma–present	chimpanzee	Brain size 350 cm^3.	Use of natural stones as tools; urge to play; display some empathy; episodic skills salient.
4–5 Ma	*Ardipithecus ramidus*	Brain size 350 cm^3.	Less aggressive than chimps· with less pronounced canine teeth; apparently lived in both trees and on ground.

3–4 Ma	*Australo-pithecus afarensis*	Brain size 475 cm^3.	Possibly split stones as tools; episodic skills salient. It's unclear if *Australopithecus* is direct ancestor of *Homo sapiens*.
1.6–2.5 Ma	*Homo habilis*	Brain size 630 cm^3.	Use of chopper tools but no teaching or innovation, tools stayed much the same for the duration of the species; mimetic skills more salient.
2 Ma–150 Ka	*Homo erectus*	Brain size 1000 cm^3.	More complex tools, like hand ax, but still no teaching or innovation within this species; speech apparatus with more clarity; mimetic skills salient.
500 Ka–28 Ka	Neanderthal	Brain size 1500 cm^3.	Even more complex tools, like spears and limited teaching and innovation; speech apparatus with more clarity; mimetic skills salient and beginnings of mythic skills.
150 Ka–present	*Homo sapiens*	Brain size 1350 cm^3.	Ever more complex tools, including ornamented knives and spears, all the way to agricultural instruments and metal weapons; much teaching and innovation through the development of human culture; speech apparatus fully developed: mythic skills fully realized.

Part II: Advances for *Homo sapiens*

125,000 Ya .... Earliest evidence of burial rituals, assuming a belief in an afterlife.

80,000 Ya .... Early art in the form of symmetrical scrapings on tools.

60,000–75,000 Ya .... Modern humans migrate out of Africa.

30,000 Ya .... Advanced cave art, modern hunting tools, more elaborate burial rituals, and evidence of musical instruments. Positive selection pressure for genes related to brain development.

10,000 Ya .... Evidence of agriculture, animal domestication, and permanent settlements. Positive selection pressure for genes related to skin color, lactate production, and, potentially, brain complexity.

6000 Ya .... Systematic written symbols appear; writing develops theoretic skills.

2000–4000 Ya .... Modern cultures in Egypt, Greece, China, Africa, and the New World.

600 Ya .... Printing press invented.

150–200 Ya .... Industrial Revolution.

50–60 Ya .... Modern computers invented.

B. Timeline of Individual Development

Developmental "Era"	Behavioral and Brain Developments
prenatal..........................	Massive neurogenesis and intial synaptogenesis; a brain at birth contains well over the adult complement of 120 billion neurons. Around 2 weeks, the neural plate develops. At 4–5 weeks, the neural tube begins to separate into hindbrain, midbrain, and forebrain, and the neural groove, forerunner of spinal cord, at 5–6 weeks. By 1–2 months the brain stem and the medial forebrain bundle begin to form. The limbic system, thalamic nuclei, and hippocampus form around 2–3 months. The cerebellum and corpus callosum form at 3–4 months. Cortical neurons form during first third of prenatal development, but particular regions migrate more slowly. Around 5 months, we respond to light, when eyes are open; and around 5–6 months we respond to sound. Myelination occurs from 7 months until well after birth, extending through adolescence in some regions; portions of prefrontal cortex are last to myelinate. Many more convolutions develop between 7–9 months in the frontal cortex, but the region does not fully mature for over 20 years.
infancy (0–1 year).........	Myelination continues rapidly, speeding up neural transmission; massive synaptogenesis and pruning. Several infant reflexes and temperamental features emerge; attachment security or insecurity develops; Piaget's sensorimotor stage of development.
toddlerhood (1–3 years)	Continuing synaptogenesis and pruning occurs; language explosion occurs.

early childhood/
preschool (4–5 years)....Theory of mind fully emerges; peer
relationships multiply; Piaget's
preoperational stage of development.

middle–late childhood
(6–10 years) ....Intensive growth of academic skills; cortical
"thinning" normatively occurs; Piaget's
concrete operational stage of development.

early adolescence
(11–15 years)..................Sexual maturation/pubertal development;
further frontal development takes place,
but cognitive skills outpace risk-taking
tendencies; Piaget's formal operational stage
of development.

late adolescence
(16–19 years) ....Push toward independence, but frontal
maturation is still not complete; myelination
finally completed in some frontal regions;
cognitive maturation; peak or near peak in
many perceptual-motor skills.

young adulthood
(20–39 years) ....Full maturation of frontal lobes; if used,
verbal skills continue to develop; new
families emerge; intimacy and commitment
issues salient; responsiveness and sensitivity
to offspring predicts security.

middle adulthood
(40–69 years) ....Gradual declines in motor skills; time of
life during which engagement in mental
and physical activities appears crucial for
maintenance of cognitive functioning.

older adulthood
(70+ years)....................Socioemotional selectivity theory (SST)
comes into play.

Glossary

Terms are defined briefly, with reference to this course; complete definitions may be beyond the scope of this glossary in many instances.

action potential: Brief electrical signal related to changes in a neuron's membrane potential; produces a nerve impulse.

additive model (of behavior genetics): The model contending that individual differences in traits or behaviors are attributable to genetic factors, shared environmental factors, and non-shared or unique environmental factors, all of which are independent of one another.

adolescence: Developmental period beginning at the time of puberty/sexual maturation; the end point is harder to pinpoint (e.g., development of independence from family of origin).

adoption studies: Method of inferring heritability in behavior genetics research, through comparing rates of a trait or disorder in biological versus adoptive relatives.

affective style: Individual's emotional tone for long periods of time, probably related to vestiges of early temperament.

agreeableness: One of the Big Five personality traits, linked to social warmth, empathy, optimism, and absence of hostility.

alleles: Variants of a given gene, with 1 form inherited from each parent.

amygdala: Almond-shaped subcortical nucleus; linked to basic emotions, especially fear.

antipsychotic medications: Psychoactive medications used to treat psychosis and schizophrenia; first-generation formulations blockade the postsynaptic dopamine receptor; second-generation formulations have more complex actions on dopamine, serotonin, and other neurotransmitters.

Ardipithecus ramidus: A primate species, living between 4 and 5 million years ago. Thought to be a forerunner of *Australopithecus afarensis* ("Lucy"); an intermediate between chimpanzees and modern hominids. Speculation is that this species lived both in trees and on the ground.

artificial intelligence (AI): Machine-based, computer intelligence. *See* **Turing test**.

Asperger's disorder: Synonymous with high-functioning autism, in which an individual has normal intelligence, yet social oddities and idiosyncratic speech dominate the clinical picture.

attachment: The naturally selected processes of parent-child bonds in primates; individual differences in human attachment are assumed to relate to parental responsiveness to infants during the first year of life.

attention: Crucial mental process, akin to a "spotlight," signaling which stimuli the individual should focus on. Important subtypes include automatic attention, selective attention, executive attention, and sustained attention.

attention-deficit/hyperactivity disorder (ADHD): Mental disorder characterized by extremes of inattention, impulsivity, and hyperactivity; originates in childhood; treated with stimulant medications and/or behavior therapy.

attribution: An individual's causal explanation for an event or occurrence.

Australopithecus afarensis: Primate species living approximately 3–4 million years ago; assumed to be a direct ancestor of hominids and modern humans, perhaps having descended from *Ardipithecus ramidus*. Lucy is the name of the complete female skeleton.

authoritarian parenting: Style marked by high levels of control/demands but low levels of warmth/responsiveness; associated with overcompliance or aggression, but not in all ethnic groups.

authoritative parenting: Style marked by high levels of both warmth/responsiveness and control/demands; associated generally with good academic and social outcomes.

autism/autistic disorder: Mental disorder with origins early in childhood, marked by social isolation, language difficulties and abnormalities, restricted play, and a need for order and sameness.

autoreceptor: Receptor for the neurotransmitter of a neuron located on the axon of that same neuron; stimulation of autoreceptor usually serves to slow synthesis of that neurotransmitter.

axon: Long "arm" of a neuron, carrying signals down its length to the synapse.

Baldwin effect: Hypothesized mechanism of natural selection in which general learning abilities are favored as adaptations.

behavior genetics: Field of study to infer genetic, or heritable, versus environmental contributions to individual differences in traits and conditions; major research methods include family studies, twin studies, and adoption studies.

behavior therapy: Application of principles of classical and/or operant conditioning to mental disorders, such as phobias, depression, ADHD, and schizophrenia.

Big Five personality traits: Commonly accepted structure of adult personality, captured by acronym OCEAN representing 5 core traits: openness to experience, conscientiousness, extraversion, agreeableness, and neuroticism.

bipolar disorder: Severe mood disorder with alternating periods of depression, mania, and mixed states (combining manic and depressive features). Highly heritable; highly associated with risk for suicide, if untreated. Formerly termed manic-depressive illness.

blindsight: The implicit ability to "see" without conscious perception of objects.

case study: Research method involving intensive investigation of a single individual; leads to rich information but may be subject to non-representativeness and lack of control of extraneous variables.

cerebellum: Large area above brain stem linked to motor coordination, timing of actions, and learning.

classical conditioning: Form of learning in which unconditioned stimuli, which trigger an involuntary response, are paired temporally with conditioned or neutral stimuli, such that the conditioned stimuli come to evoke the initial response.

cognition: Processes of thinking; specifically, in cognitive science, refers to information processing models of the mind.

cognitive-behavioral therapy/cognitive therapy: Updated versions of behavior therapy, whereby cognitive processes and not just learned behaviors are the subject of active modification.

cognitive control: *See* **executive functions.**

cognitive map: Tolman's concept that even mice and rats learn a maze form a visualization of the maze; thus, learning can occur without reinforcement.

cognitive psychology: Product of cognitive revolution of the 1950s and beyond, the study of mental processes as underlying much of human behavior: perception, memory, higher-order abstract thinking, and the like.

concrete operational stage of development: Third stage of Piaget's model of cognitive development when children become able to reason logically about concrete events and objects, approximate ages 7–12.

connectivity: Patterns of synaptic linkages in the brain; high levels of connectivity are found in human brains.

conscientiousness: One of the Big Five personality traits, linked to achievement-orientation, carefulness, reliability, and deliberation.

consciousness: Subjective awareness, knowledge of self, and meta-awareness—that is, awareness of one's awareness; the subject of renewed scientific efforts related to gaining an understanding of how human self-awareness evolved.

correlational research: Method of appraising whether one variable is associated with another; commonly used in research on the human mind, when experimental control is not possible.

cortex: The outermost layers of our cerebral hemispheres; also known a "grey matter" because of accumulations of cell nuclei.

cranium: The skull; fossilized craniums are essential for inferring brain size.

critical period: Developmental "window" during which, if a psychological process does not take place, it will be too late afterwards. *Contrast with* **sensitive period**.

cultural evolution: Processes, in recent human history, of gains in human skill through means other than natural selection.

culture: A system of shared beliefs and values, transmitted by social groups to their members, shaping and guiding perceptions and behavior.

defense mechanisms: In psychoanalytic theory, the unconscious mental processes that mask the underlying conflicts, to ward off anxiety. Examples include denial, repression, projection, introjection, and sublimation.

delusion: A fixed, false belief that is extremely resistant to rational argument; a symptom of psychosis.

dendrite: Postsynaptic end of neuron; receives chemical input from axon terminal of presynaptic neuron via receptors.

depression: Mood disorder marked by a sad mood, despair, cognitive distortions, hopelessness, sleep and appetite disturbance, and suicidal thoughts; episodes tend to repeat across the lifespan.

depressive realism: Tendency for individuals with depression to not show positive illusory bias, with grim but accurate perceptions of personal deficits.

developmental gene: A gene that activates key processes during prenatal or early childhood phases of life, triggering a cascade of developmental processes. *See also* **evo-devo**.

developmental psychopathology: Field of study integrating normal developmental processes and atypical behavior patterns.

diffusion tensor imaging (DTI): An imaging technique allowing appraisal of the white-matter tracts of the brain; used to infer connectivity.

disorganized attachment: Individual difference in attachment security; child has no consistent response to parent's return after absence, engaging in disconnected, freezing behavior; believe to result from frightening, abusive parental behavior.

DNA (deoxyribonucleic acid): Complex double-helical molecule, found in the nucleus of every cell, that contains the genetic code for life; divided into chromosomes, genes, and non-genetic material.

dopamine: Key neurotransmitter related to attention, reward, voluntary motor movement, and higher cognitive function.

dualism: Belief that mind and body are different entities, which cannot be reduced to each other.

effortful control: Temperamental characteristic emerging near the end of the first year of life, related to increasing ability to regulate attention and sustain attempts to manipulate the environment.

emotion: Action tendency and feeling state, motivating and organizing an organism; composed of physiological, subjective, and facial components; a number of basic positive and negative emotions have been identified cross-culturally.

emotion regulation: Means of modulating or responding to one's emotions; major subtypes include reappraisal of emotion-eliciting situations or suppression of emotion displays. Begins during the first year of life as self-soothing; becomes increasingly sophisticated with maturation of frontal lobes and internalization of social input.

empathy: The sharing or matching of emotions with another person; subdivisions include emotional empathy or emotion matching and cognitive empathy.

empiricism: Philosophical contention that knowledge emanates from experience and evidence; thus, the mind is a blank slate at birth, with learning accounting for the human mind.

epigenetic factors: Broadly speaking, changes in gene expression for reasons other than actual alterations of genetic code.

episodic skills: First stage of prehuman cognitive development, per Merlin Donald, in which extensive memories guide adaptive behavior.

evo-devo (the evolution of development): Subfield of evolutionary theory dealing with genes expressed early in development, even prenatally; such genes alter developmental processes to create novel structures and functions. More generally, the field of study of the origin of developmental processes in all life forms.

evolution: Based on natural selection, a model developed by Darwin on the origin of diversity, and of species, among life forms.

evolutionary psychology: Field of study that views human traits as adaptations, subject to natural selection, or sexual selection; such universal tendencies interacting with culture and to shape specific behavior patterns in an individual.

executive functions: High-level mental processes subserved by the frontal lobes and their extensive connectivity with other brain regions, including planning, monitoring performance, inhibiting extraneous mental processes, and correcting errors.

experiment: Research method involving the random assignment of subjects to conditions, so that causal inferences are best made.

extinction: In psychology, form of operant conditioning in which response is followed by no stimulus, decreasing subsequent frequency of response. In evolution, the dying out of a species.

extraversion: One of the Big Five personality traits, linked to gregariousness, assertiveness, energy level, and tendencies toward action as opposed to reflection.

family (pedigree) studies: Method of determining heritability in behavior genetics research, through correlating degree of relatedness of family members with their risk of developing a certain condition or disorder; subject to the confound that more closely related individuals tend to share more interpersonal contact.

formal operational stage of development: Fourth stage of Piaget's model of cognitive development when youth become able to think abstractly and hypothetically; approximate ages 12 and up.

frontal lobe: Region of the cortex above the eyes and back toward the middle of the skull; larger in primates than other animals; linked to planning and emotional behavior.

functional magnetic resonance imaging (fMRI): Computer-assisted brain scanning device that uses powerful magnets to track oxygen levels in various brain regions; has the ability to track where neural activity has recently occurred.

gamma-amino butyric acid (GABA): Major inhibitory neurotransmitter in the brain.

gender: Psychologically and culturally determined differences between males and females. *See also* **sex**.

gene: Unit of DNA on a given chromosome that codes for a particular protein..

gene-environment correlation: The linking of genetic influences on traits or behaviors with contextual influences; such association may be passive, whereby children's environments are correlated with the genes inherited from parents; active, whereby children seek environments consistent with their genetically mediated traits; or evocative, whereby children elicit responses from the environment that promote their genetically-mediated tendencies.

gene-environment interaction: Process whereby certain genotypes are maximally expressed only in specific environments; reveals that "main effects" of genes or environments are often not sufficient to explain individual differences in behavior.

genotype: Genetic make-up of organism; particular allelic combination underlying a given trait or behavior.

glial cell: Support cells to neurons in the brain; source of myelin.

goodness of fit: The matching of caregiving style to a child's temperament; evidence exists that more than temperament alone or caregiving alone, the fit is essential for optimal development.

grey matter: Brain areas with an accumulation of cell bodies; characterizes the cortical layers of the brain.

hallucination: Perception in the absence of a stimulus (e.g., hearing voices, seeing visions); symptom of psychosis.

hemisphere: One of the 2 major divisions of the brain; typically, the right is specialized for spatial functions and the left for language functions.

heritability: Proportion of variation in a trait or behavior attributable to genes, rather than environments.

heterozygote superiority: The adaptive success of an organism with 2 different alleles.

hippocampus: Brain structure found in temporal lobe essential for consolidation of long-term memories.

hominids: Species of the genus *Homo*, originating 2.5 million years ago; the only surviving species is our own species, *Homo sapiens*.

Homo sapiens (*Homo sapiens sapiens*): Our species, originating approximately 150,000 years ago in Africa, and which has undergone extensive microevolution and cultural evolution since its inception, creating the modern human mind.

humanism: The perspective that the mind is linked to universal human processes and values, with the creation of narrative a key feature.

implicit mental processes: Mental processes occurring beneath conscious awareness, including attitudes, perception, and memory.

inhibitory control: The ability to suppress a previously-rewarded response, freeing the organism from constraints of the immediate environment.

insecure attachment: Individual difference in attachment security; insecure attachment comes in the form of avoidant attachment or ambivalent/resistant attachment; both believed to emerge from less-than responsive parenting during initial months of life.

instinct: In biological psychology, an inherited, fixed disposition toward behavior that does not require learning (or very little learning) to become fully formed. Although it is often assumed that humans have very few instincts compared to most other species—because of human neural plasticity and learning capacity—evolutionary psychologists contend that humans actually have a host of instinctive, automatic mental modules.

joint (shared) attention: The following of a gaze or a "point" by child and parent; severely compromised in young children with autism.

learning: Acquisition of knowledge, behavior, skills, values, and the like, through classical or operant conditioning or modeling.

levels of analysis: The spanning of genes, gene products, neurons, and brains through the contextual influences on factors such as families, schools, neighborhoods, and cultures, leading to a constant interplay across such factors.

magnetic resonance imaging (MRI; known as structural MRI): Computer-assisted brain scanning in which strong magnetic fields provide anatomical pictures of soft tissue.

manic-depressive illness: *See* **bipolar disorder**.

meme: Hypothesized unit of cultural transmission; an idea or concept, spread via human communication, which may be subject to an analogue of natural selection.

mental illness (models of mental illness): Dysfunctional behavioral and emotional patterns yielding high levels of impairment and personal suffering; underlying models include statistical, social deviance, moral, ecological/impairment, medical, harmful dysfunction, and developmental psychopathology.

mental synthesis: Creation of never-before-seen mental images from previous perspectives or images; per Andrey Vyshedskiy, this is one of the few uniquely human capacities.

mimetic skills: Second phase of hominid development, per Merlin Donald, in which imitative skills formed the basis of learning and cultural transmission; associated with pre-humans.

mind: The total set of mental processes, linked intimately with brain functioning.

modeling: Form of social learning in which behavior is learned through observation of model, without reinforcement.

module (mental): Specific, innate program of the mind, instinctive, guiding cognitive or social processes. Modules are assumed to be units of mental processing that evolved in response to various selection pressures.

monoamine oxidase (MAO): Enzyme inside the presynaptic axon terminal that may degrade neurotransmitters that are not inside vesicles.

monoamine-oxidase inhibitor: Monoamine-oxidase inhibitors are medications that break down MAO, leading to higher functional levels of the neurotransmitter.

mood: Affective state lasting longer than a discrete emotion, spanning minutes or hours.

mutation: Error in DNA sequence produced during copying; often harmful, but could lead to diversity that is adaptive.

myelin: Fatty sheath or coating around axons, greatly increasing conduction speed; formed from oligodendrocyte glial cells.

mythic skills: Third phase of hominid development, per Merlin Donald, in which spoken language became the main means of communication and cultural transmission; associated with modern humans.

narrative: A means of communication involving stories with sequences of events; narratives are a common means of transmitting culture.

nativism (innatism): Philosophical contention that the mind is guided by inborn processes and instincts.

natural experiment: A means of inferring causal relationships between events when full randomization is not possible but through natural events that juxtapose causal factors.

natural selection: The process through which evolution works: Mutations may lead to structures or traits producing fitness for reproduction, propagating such genes in future generations; hence, nature "selects" such genes.

naturalism: The perspective that the mind is the result of observable physical processes; directly juxtaposed to spirit-based views.

nature versus nurture: Outmoded juxtaposition of biological/genetic verses psychosocial influences on human development; such influences work in concert, rather than in opposition.

negative reinforcement: Form of operant conditioning in which response is followed by cessation of aversive stimulus, increasing subsequent frequency of response.

neglectful parenting: Style marked by low levels of both warmth/responsiveness and control/demands; associated with extremely poor cognitive and social outcomes.

neural correlates of consciousness: Brain regions, neural tracts, and neural processes that are associated with human self-awareness and sentience through brain imaging and other techniques.

neuroethics: Subfield at the conjunction of neuroscience and ethics dealing with brain mechanisms underlying human ethics and ethical implications of advances in neuroscience.

neurogenesis: Process of formation of neurons; most neurogenesis is prenatal in origin.

neuron: Specialized cell of the brain and nervous system; contains dendrites, cell body, and axons; conducts electrical current.

neuroticism: One of the Big Five personality traits, linked to pessimism, proneness to anxiety, stress reactivity, and becoming overwhelmed.

neurotransmitter: Chemical released from presynaptic axon terminal, traversing synaptic cleft to interact with postsynaptic receptor on a dendrite.

non-shared (unique) environment: The set of environmental factors that are not shared by children in the same family (e.g., peers; different parental styles with different children).

norepinephrine: Major neurotransmitter, related to appetite, sleep/wake cycles, impulse control, blood flow, and more.

obsessive-compulsive disorder (OCD): Mental disorder characterized by unwanted, ruminative thoughts (obsessions) and repetitive behaviors that attempt to undo the obsessions (compulsions).

occipital lobe: Region of the cortex at the back of the skull; linked particularly to vision.

ontogeny: The individual's developmental course from fertilized egg through maturity.

openness to experience: One of the Big Five personality traits, linked to appreciation of the arts, intellectual curiosity, and deeply-felt emotions.

operant conditioning: Form of learning whereby responses of the organism are followed by stimuli that either increase or decrease the subsequent probability of responding. The 4 types are positive reinforcement, punishment, negative reinforcement, and extinction.

parietal lobe: Region of the cortex from the top of the skull back toward the occipital lobe; linked to sensory functions and motor functions.

perception: The active processes involved in gaining access to constructs in the world through the sensory organs.

permissive parenting: Style marked by high levels of warmth/responsiveness but low levels of control/demands; associated generally with lowered academic outcomes.

personality: Overall structure of person's cognitive, social, and behavioral features; formed from combinations of core personality traits. *See* **Big Five personality traits**.

phenotype: Observable characteristics, traits, or behaviors or an organism; expression of genotype, epigenetic factors, and environments working in concert.

phrenology: Pseudoscience of the 19th century, contending that personality is shaped by brain anatomy, able to be "read" by patterns of bumps on the skull.

phylogeny: The domain of evolutionary processes, across species from early times on Earth until the present.

plasticity: Changes in brain function and structure related to experience; human brains have been naturally selected for a great amount of plasticity.

positive illusory bias: Everyday set of cognitive distortions in which normally functioning individuals underapprise personal weaknesses and overestimate personal abilities.

positive reinforcement: Form of operant conditioning in which response is followed by rewarding stimulus, increasing subsequent frequency of response.

positron emission tomography (PET): Method of imaging body or brain using radioactive substances to examine metabolism and activity.

post-traumatic stress disorder (PTSD): Mental disorder linked to overwhelming trauma, characterized by re-experiencing of the event, numbing, and physiological overreactivity.

preoperational stage of development: Second stage of Piaget's model of cognitive development where children come to represent and express experiences in language and symbolic thought; approximate 2–7 years of age.

primates: Class of species originating 80 million years ago, including monkeys, great apes, hominids, and humans.

priming: In cognitive psychology, the process in which an early stimulus influences responses to later stimuli.

protective factor: Variable that occurs in the presence of a risk factor to mitigate the risk or vulnerability, promoting resilience.

pruning: Selective loss of neurons that do not form viable synapses with other neurons; necessary for optimal brain development.

psychoanalysis: Form of therapy originated by Freud; intensive, daily treatment in which the patient discusses dreams and free associates, with the therapist interpreting the unconscious material.

psychoanalytic/psychodynamic theory: Theoretical models of the mind, derived from Freud (psychoanalytic) or successors (psychodynamic) emphasizing unconscious motivation, defense mechanisms, and parent-child conflict in explaining behavior.

psychosis: Syndrome involving hallucinations, delusions, agitation, thought disorder, loss of contact with reality.

punishment: Form of operant conditioning in which response is followed by aversive stimulus, decreasing subsequent frequency of response.

qualia: Subjective quality of a percept or experience; not believed to be reducible to brain chemistry or other naturalistic phenomena.

reciprocal altruism: Pattern of sharing resources without immediate benefit, in the hope of receiving subsequent "payback"; may be a core mechanism of human social bonds.

reciprocal determinism: Process of individual development whereby individual characteristics affect environment at the same time that environment affects individual.

resilience: The processes whereby an individual at high risk develops better than expected outcomes; often attributed to the presence of protective factors.

reuptake: Process of reabsorption of neurotransmitters into presynaptic regions; linked to transporter molecules.

risk factor: Variable that precedes a negative outcome and correlates with that outcome.

schizophrenia: Mental disorder involving positive or excess symptoms and negative or deficit symptoms; often extremely debilitating.

secure attachment: Pattern of child's being soothed by parental return after separation and using parent as secure base for exploration; believed to emerge from responsive parenting during initial months of life.

self-esteem: Inner sense of self-worth.

Self-organization: The process whereby the internal organization of a system (like a brain, or a mind) increases in complexity without explicit external guidance.

sensitive period: Developmental "window" during which learning or development optimally takes place, although some learning may occur outside that window. *Contrast with* **critical period**.

sensorimotor stage of development: First stage of Piaget's model of cognitive development, in which infants and toddlers express intelligence through sensory and motor functions and abilities; occuring from birth to approximately 2 years of age.

serotonin (5-HT): Neurotransmitter involved in emotional responses, sleep, and many other functions.

serotonin-selective reuptake inhibitors (SSRIs): Used in the treatment of depression and anxiety, these medications block the serotonin transporter, allowing more serotonin in the synaptic cleft.

sex: Biological maleness or femaleness, determined by genes and prenatal hormonal influences.

sexual selection: Form of natural selection in which differential tasks or problems encountered by males verses females lead to differentiation of physical structures and behaviors. In intrasexual selection, males fight among themselves for access to females; in intersexual selection, females choose for preferred males.

shared environment: The set of environmental factors that are shared by children in the same family (e.g., parenting styles, income levels).

social learning theory: The modern combination of behaviorism, modeling, and additional cognitive processes, based on the conception that most human behavior is learned.

sociobiology: Field originated by E. O. Wilson in 1970s dealing with naturally selected bases of social behavior; forerunner of evolutionary psychology.

socioemotional selectivity theory (SST): Theoretical model that as people age, they develop foreshortened time horizons leading to the accentuation of positive emotions and the display of emotional wisdom.

sociometric status: The level of peer approval or disapproval one receives, based on nominations of being liked or disliked from the peer group. Children may be popular, average, neglected, rejected, or controversial where they are liked by some and disliked by others.

stigma: Internal mark of shame, related to membership in a devalued social group; composed of stereotypes, prejudice, and discrimination.

stimulant medications: Used in the treatment of ADHD, these medications block the reuptake of dopamine and norepinephrine, increasing attentional focus and enhancing inhibitory control.

strange situation: Assessment method for appraising an infant's attachment security; involves caregiver and stranger entering and exiting room with infant.

synaptogenesis: Process of formation of synaptic connections between and among neurons; driven by genetic programs and experience; reaches a peak in the first years of life.

synapse: Junction between neurons; composed of preysnaptic axon terminal, synaptic cleft (space in between), and postsynaptic dendritic spines. Neurotransmitters cross the cleft to communicate between neurons.

temperament: Early appearing, biologically determined emotional and behavioral response tendencies; aspects of temperament form the basis of later personality.

temporal lobe: Region of the cortex above the ear, or temple; linked to hearing, language, and memory.

tertiary regions (association areas): Portions of cortex that do not receive direct sensory input but rather make abstract connections between concepts; these regions are larger in humans than other primates.

thalamus: Subcortical region; "relay station" of sensory inputs to the cortex.

theoretic skills: Fourth phase of hominid development, per Merlin Donald, in which written language became the main means of communication and cultural transmission; associated with extremely modern humans.

theory of mind: Mental module assumed to come "online" between 3–5 years of age, through which children come to the understanding that other humans have perspectives different from their own.

thought disorder (formal): Disturbance in the structure and form of thinking and speech processes; symptom of psychosis and schizophrenia.

toolkit gene: Gene that regulates the actions of other genes; also called "master gene."

tract: Nerve pathway, composed of axons traversing different brain regions.

transporter: Molecule that facilitates reuptake of neurotransmitter back into presynaptic region.

Turing test: "Test" suggested by mathematician Alan Turing for appraising the success of artificial intelligence, as measured by whether a conversation with a computer versus a conversation with a human would be indistinguishable.

twin studies: Method of inferring heritability in behavior genetics research, through determining the difference in concordance rates of a trait or disorder between identical versus fraternal twins.

unconscious mental processes: Cognitive and emotional activities that transpire without awareness. In cognitive psychology, unconscious processes are often termed implicit (unaware) attitudes, perceptions, and memory; in psychoanalytic theory, the unconscious is a conflict-ridden terrain at the intersection of the id, ego, and superego.

vesicles: Storage areas in presynaptic axon terminals, protecting neurotransmitters from enzymatic degradation.

white matter: Axonal regions of neurons; appear white because of myelination; source of connectivity of brain.

Biographical Notes

These are very brief sketches of a few key individuals, throughout history, who have contributed to our knowledge of the origins of the human mind. The large numbers of contemporary neuroscientists, evolutionary biologists, evolutionary psychologists, and other scientists who are interested in and contributing to this topic cannot be noted here.

Bowlby, John (1907–1990): British psychiatrist who brought attachment theory to scientific and public attention. His early work on institutionalized infants, delinquency, and poor childrearing practices culminated, in mid- and late career, with seminal work on the species-wide importance of attachment, drawing from a diversity of fields: evolution, ethology, developmental psychology, and cognitive science. His thinking on attachment integrated evolutionary theory, psychodynamic theory, and developmental studies. His major 3-volume set on attachment theory includes *Attachment* (1969), *Separation: Anxiety and Anger* (1972), and *Loss: Sadness and Depression* (1980).

Chomsky, Noam (1928–): American linguist, philosopher, cognitive scientist, and political activist/dissident; Chomsky contributed greatly to the cognitive revolution and to "innatist" views of the human mind in his early psycholinguistic work, during the 1950s, in which he critiqued B. F. Skinner's operant conditioning account of language development and posited a fixed, innate, universal grammar underlying all human languages. Over the years he has become known as much for his radical political views as his work in cognitive science and linguistics, though he claims that the endeavors are entirely separate.

Darwin, Charles (1809–1882): One of the scientific giants in all of history, he is credited as the co-originator of the theory of evolution by natural selection. Having abandoned medical and clerical studies, this English naturalist embarked upon a 5-year, around-the-world journey on the HMS *Beagle* from 1831–1836, spending much of his time on land to make detailed observations of geological formations and a variety of species of life. After years of deliberation, and spurred by Wallace's formulation of natural selection, Darwin published *On the Origin of Species* in 1859, which became a changing point in the history of humanity's views of life, and itself as a species. Subsequent books included *The Descent of Man and Selection in Relation to Sex* (1871) and *The Expression of the Emotions in Man and Animals* (1872).

Dawkins, Richard (b. 1941): British evolutionary biologist, who has received much acclaims for his popular science writing, he wrote *The Selfish Gene* in 1976, arguing that genes are the unit of natural selection; he also introduced the concept of memes in this work. His book, *The Blind Watchmaker* in 1982, is a strong call to resist any sort of intelligent design as an explanation for the complexity of life. *The God Delusion* (2006) lays out his strongest arguments as an atheist and as a critic of creationism.

Ekman, Paul (b. 1934): American psychologist most recognized for his cross-cultural investigations of the universality of emotional displays and the universality of recognition of basic emotions. His work went against the grain of the cultural determinists of the mid-20th century. He has done extensive work on facial displays of emotion and the detection of lies. Among his books are *Emotions Revealed* (2003) and *Telling Lies* (2001).

Freud, Sigmund (1856–1939): Austrian psychiatrist and founder of psychoanalytic theory and psychoanalysis as an intensive form of psychotherapy. After studying neurology and advocating physical bases of mental disorders, Freud began to develop a completely psychological theory of normal and atypical development, based heavily on unconscious mental processes, defense mechanisms, symbolic meaning of symptoms, and inevitable conflict between individuals and society. Psychoanalytic theory was further developed by many followers; less doctrinaire versions are known as psychodynamic formulations. His work changed the way modern societies think about the mind, even though many psychoanalytic principles and concepts have not withstood empirical scrutiny.

Hippocrates (c. 460 B.C.E.–c. 375 B.C.E.): Ancient Athenian physician, known as the father of medicine, Hippocrates integrated philosophy and medicine and discredited the predominant view of the time that supernatural forces were the dominant contributors to illness. He therefore presented a completely naturalistic view of human health and illness, based on the 4 "humors"—yellow bile, black bile, blood, phlegm—and their relative balance in the body. He promoted the view that the practice of medicine should incorporate discipline, humility, professionalism, and ethics. His observations of physical and mental disorders are remarkably modern in their detail.

Mendel, Gregor (1822–1884): European priest and scientist, known as the father of modern genetics, he worked out the laws of inheritance from his investigations on pea plants in his monastery's garden. His findings were obscure until they were rediscovered after his death; in the 20th century, a major synthesis of Darwinian evolution and Mendelian genetics took place, setting the stage for the resurgence of modern evolutionary theory.

Pavlov, Ivan (1849–1936): Russian physiologist, physician, and psychologist, he discovered the essential mechanisms of classical conditioning. He won the Nobel Prize in 1904 for his work on the physiology of the digestive system; his psychological work originated from his having noticed that dogs began to salivate prior to presentation of food, at the sound of a signal. He was interested in the implications of the "conditioned reflex" for mental disorder.

Piaget, Jean (1896–1980): Swiss natural scientist and philosopher; originator of "genetic epistemology," the study of the development of knowledge of the world. Many of his theoretical ideas emanated from careful observation of his 3 children. He posited a complex theory of cognitive development, which emerges in stages throughout childhood as the result of children's active manipulation of the world. Each stage represents a new level of complexity. His books include *The Child's Conception of the World* (1928), *The Moral Judgment of the Child* (1932), *The Origins of Intelligence in Children* (1952), and *The Child's Construction of Reality* (1955).

Skinner, B. F. (1904–1990): American psychologist self-identified as a radical behaviorist, who denied any meditational properties of the mind, instead concentrating on schedules of reinforcement in relation to the learning and performance of behavior. He invented the operant conditioning chamber as a graduate student and performed considerable research on the power of such reinforcement schedules (related to operant conditioning). His book, *Verbal Behavior* (1957), served as the stimulus for Noam Chomsky's critique related to innate language structures in the human mind. Other books include *Walden Two* (1948) and *Beyond Freedom and Dignity* (1971).

Tolman, Edward Chace (1886–1959): American psychologist, who transcended the behaviorist and social learning traditions of mid-20th-century behavioral science to posit that even rats running mazes had cognitive maps and that learning could occur without reinforcement. He was a forerunner of the cognitive revolution of the 1950s and beyond. His major contributions came in journal articles and in his book, *Purposive Behavior in Animals and Men* (1932). A professor at the University of California, Berkeley, he refused to sign the state's loyalty oath during the McCarthy era, and his lawsuit led to the overturning of the oath.

Wilson. E. O. (b. 1929): American naturalist and biologist who originated the field of sociobiology—now known as evolutionary psychology. A world expert on such social species as ants, Wilson has also been an ardent advocate of preserving all species on Earth. He is a secular humanist who contends that religious activity has been naturally selected among humans. A Pulitzer-Prize winning author, he has written many books, including *Sociobiology* (1975), *On Human Nature* (1979), *The Ants* (1990), *The Diversity of Life* (1992), *Naturalist* (1994), and *Consilience* (1998).

Bibliography

Andreasen, N. C. *Brave New Brain: Conquering Mental Illness in the Era of the Genome*. New York: Oxford University Press, 2001. Readable and compelling work on brain science in relation to mental illness.

Baron-Cohen, S. *The Essential Differences*. New York: Basic Books, 2003. Engaging exploration of sexual differentiation of the human brain and human behavior.

Beardslee, W. *Out of the Darkened Room*. Boston: Little, Brown, 2002. Compelling account of the author's model of therapy for families in which a parent has a mood disorder; emphasizes the importance of creating a family narrative for enhancing children's coping.

Beauchaine, T., and S. P. Hinshaw, eds. *Child Psychopathology*. Hoboken, NJ: Wiley, 2008. Edited compendium of recent research on the origins and manifestations of child and adolescent mental disorders, with emphasis on psychobiology and gene-environment interactions.

Bloom, P. *Descartes' Baby*. New York: Basic Books, 2004. Intriguing account of childhood, social development, and their linkages to evolutionary theory.

Bowlby, J. *A Secure Base: Parent-Child Attachment and Healthy Human Development*. New York: Basic Books, 1988. Compact and readable account of the implications of attachment for developmental outcomes, into adulthood.

Brizendine, L. *The Female Brain*. New York: Morgan Hill Books, 2006. Intriguing, if sometimes overstated, view of biological differences between male and female brains and behavior patterns.

Buss, D. *The Evolution of Desire: Strategies of Human Mating*. New York: Basic Books, 2003. Evolutionary psychological account of sexual selection and human courtship and mating strategies.

———. *Evolutionary Psychology: The New Science of the Mind*. Boston: Allyn & Bacon, 2004. Popularized account of the field of evolutionary psychology; doesn't shrink from controversy.

Damasio, A. *Descartes' Error*. New York: Avon, 1994. Discusses dualism, reasoning, emotion, and the brain, in the author's typically engaging style.

Dawkins, R. *River Out of Eden: A Darwinian View of Life*. New York: Basic Books, 1995. Compelling account of modern implications of evolutionary theory.

———. *The Selfish Gene*. New York: Oxford University Press, 2006. Newest edition of the author's classic work on his view of how evolution works at the level of gene selection.

Deacon, T. W. *The Symbolic Species: The Co-Evolution of Language and the Brain*. New York: Norton, 1997. Scholarly work on human language abilities, their natural selection, and linkages with brain development.

Dennett, D. C. *Consciousness Explained*. New York: Little, Brown, 1991. Eloquent argument that consciousness is not what most believe it to be; a bit out of date, but provocative.

Donald, M. *A Mind So Rare: The Evolution of Human Consciousness*. New York: Norton, 2001. Treatise contending that reductionist notions of modular human minds cannot explain the full power of the mind outside of laboratory studies; eloquent and compelling.

———. *Origins of the Modern Mind*. Cambridge: Harvard University Press, 1991. The author's original exposition of evolution of minds from episodic to mimetic to mythic to theoretic. Readable and intriguing.

Dukakis, K. *Shock: The Healing Power of Electroconvulsive Therapy*. New York: Avery, 2006. Vivid first-person account of the author's deep depressions and substance abuse issues and of the therapeutic benefits of ECT.

Edelman, G. *Wider than the Sky*. New Haven: Yale University Press, 2004. Account of human consciousness written by Nobel-Prize winning scientist.

Ekman, P. *Emotions Revealed*. New York: Henry Holt, 2003. Popular book about emotions, their universality, their expressions, and their blends.

Gazzaniga, M. *The Ethical Brain*. New York: Dana Press, 2005. Which areas of the brain are involved in ethical and moral behavior? This is the subject of this accessible and scholarly book.

———. *Human: The Science Behind What Makes Us Unique*. New York: HarperCollins, 2008. Comprehensive, complex, yet readable book on human reasoning, emotion, social behavior, etc., and evolutionary forces that have driven human qualities.

Goffman, E. *Stigma: Notes on the Management of Spoiled Identity*. Englewood Cliffs, NJ: Prentice-Hall, 1963. This slender volume is a classic on the concept of stigma, written by the eminent sociologist.

Gottesman, I. *Schizophrenia Genesis*. New York: Freeman, 1991. Readable and compelling overview of the manifestations and causes of schizophrenia, including a number of first-person accounts.

Grandin, T. *Thinking in Pictures*. New York: Doubleday, 1995. Written by a scientist with high-functioning autism, this is an intriguing first-person account.

Hinshaw, S. P., ed. *Breaking the Silence*. New York: Oxford University Press, 2008. Compilation of first-person and family accounts of mental disorder, from mental health professionals.

———. *The Mark of Shame: Stigma of Mental Illness and an Agenda for Change*. New York: Oxford University Press, 2007. Comprehensive account of the tendencies for humans to castigate and discriminate against fellow humans with mental disorders.

———. *The Triple Bind: Saving our Teenage Girls from Today's Pressures* . Discusses cultural reasons for the alarming rates of increase in teenage girls' rates of mental disorder in recent years.

———. *The Years of Silence are Past: My Father's Life with Bipolar Disorder*. New York: Cambridge University Press, 2002. Biographical and autobiographical account of the life of the course instructor's father (and himself).

Jamison, K. R. *An Unquiet Mind*. New York: Vintage, 1995. Moving personal account of bipolar disorder by the Johns Hopkins psychologist, a former supervisor of the course instructor.

Julien, R. M. *A Primer of Drug Action*. New York: Freeman, 2001. Basic, thorough tour of pharmacokinetics, pharmacodynamics, and mechanisms of action of medications on mental illnesses.

King, B. *Evolving God*. New York: Doubleday, 2007. From the perspective of an expert in primatology, this book examines the deep bonds between primate infants and caregivers as the ultimate basis of belongingness and religious belief. The book is, however, extremely dismissive of any evolutionary/genetic bases of religious belief.

Kring, A., and S. L. Johnson. *Abnormal Psychology*. 11th ed. Hoboken, NJ: Wiley, 2010. Latest edition of a classic textbook on mental disorders and abnormal psychology.

Koch, C. *The Quest for Consciousness*. Englewood, CO: Roberts & Company. Major discussion of human consciousness.

Kramer, P. D. *Listening to Prozac*. New York: Viking, 1995. A modern classic, one of the first popular book discussions of the new generation of antidepressant medications, introducing the concept of "cosmetic psychopharmacology."

Nasar, S. *A Beautiful Mind*. New York: Simon & Schuster, 1998. The biography of Nobel-Prize winning game theorist John Nash, whose life with schizophrenia was documented in the film of the same name.

Nigg, J. T. *What Causes ADHD?* New York: Guilford Press, 2006. Thorough compendium of causal factors for ADHD, written by world expert.

Ochs, E., and L. Capps. *Living Narrative: Creating Lives in Everyday Storytelling*. Cambridge: Harvard University Press, 2001. Major work on the use of narrative in our species, including the creation of self through life narratives.

Pies, R. W. *Handbook of Essential Psychopharmacology*. 2nd ed. Washington, D.C.: American Psychiatric Press, 2005. Filled with tables and "Q & A" sections, this is an authoritative guide to medications for the treatment of mental illness.

Pinker, S. *How the Mind Works*. New York: Norton, 1997. Superb and witty book on the workings of the mind, from a modern evolutionary psychology perspective.

————. *The Language Instinct*. New York: Harper, 1995. Another superb book, this one on the instinctive features of all human languages.

Ramachandran, V. S. *A Brief Tour of Human Consciousness: From Imposter Poodles to Purple Numbers*. New York: PI Press, 2004. Readable and provocative case studies of neurological anomalies and their implications for consciousness.

Ridley, M. *Genome: The Autobiography of a Species in 23 Chapters*. New York: Perennial, 1999. Extremely readable account of the new era of human genetics, from a noted science writer.

Rizzolatti, G., and C. Sinigaglia. *Mirrors in the Brain: How our Minds Share Actions and Emotions*. Oxford, UK: Oxford University Press, 2008. Fascinating discussion of mirror neurons, written by the Italian research group who were among the initial discoverers of these types of neurons.

Sacks, O. *An Anthropologist on Mars*. New York: Knopf, 1995. Compendium of fascinating and at times moving essays on individuals with various neurological and mental disorders.

————. *The Man Who Mistook his Wife for a Hat*. London: Chester Music, 1996. More essays (many of which originally appeared in the New York Review of Books) and case studies of neurological disorders, written in engaging and compassionate style.

Searle, J. R. *The Mystery of Consciousness*. New York: New York Review of Books, 1997. Essays from the master philosopher on human consciousness.

Siegler, R., Deloache, J., and N. Eisenberg. *How Children Develop*. New York: Worth, 2003. Wonderful textbook on child development; richly detailed yet readable.

Sigman, M., & Capps, L. Children with Autism: A Developmental Perspective. Cambridge: Harvard University Press, 1997. Scholarly yet accessible account of the ways in which autism reflects deviations in normal developmental processes.

Solomon, A. *The Noonday Demon: An Atlas of Depression*. New York: Scribner, 2001. Harrowing, insightful first-person account of severe depression.

Solomon, R. C. *True to our Feelings*. New York: Oxford University Press, 2007. Fascinating account of how emotions enrich all of our lives.

Styron, W. *Darkness Visible*. New York: Vintage, 1990. Brief, deeply moving personal narrative of life-threatening depression, eloquently written by the author, an eminent novelist.

Thornicroft, G. *Shunned: Discrimination Against People with Mental Illness*. New York: Oxford University Press, 2006. Scholarly and moving account of mental illness stigma.

Vyshedskiy, A. *On the Origin of the Human Mind*. MobileReference, 2008. Complex yet brief book on mental synthesis and the evolution from primates through hominids related to unique human mental abilities.

Wilson, E. O. *Consilience: The Unity of Knowledge*. New York: Knopf, 1998. Eloquent plea from renowned naturalist for unification of humanities, social sciences, and natural sciences.

Whybrow, P. C. *A Mood Apart: Depression, Mania, and Other Afflictions of the Self*. New York: Basic Books, 1997. Excellent synthesis of clinical and scientific literatures on mood disorders.

Wright, R. *The Evolution of God*. Boston: Little Brown, 2009. Stunning book on human conceptions of higher powers, with the thesis that more compassionate deities have "evolved" with societal changes since recorded history.

Notes

Notes